WORK HARDENING

A Practical Guide

D1552298

WORK HARDENING

A Practical Guide

Linda M. Demers, PT

Miliken Physical Therapy Center
Scarborough, Maine

Andover Medical Publishers
Boston London Oxford Singapore Sydney Toronto Wellington

Andover Medical Publishers is an imprint of Butterworth-Heinemann.

Library of Congress Catalog Card Number: 92-81340
ISBN 1-56372-022-1

Butterworth-Heinemann
80 Montvale Avenue
Stoneham, MA 02180

10 9 8 7 6 5 4 3 2 1

Printed in the United States of America

CONTENTS

PREFACE

Throughout my early involvement with the work-injured population, I found myself frustrated with the lack of useful, basic information upon which to build an effective work-hardening program. As with all new fields, there is usually a trial-and-error period to determine what works and what does not. Because we, as professionals, start with a certain body of knowledge, eventually a successful plan of action is implemented. The purpose of this publication is to provide that baseline body of knowledge in one concise reference.

It will become clear early on in your perusal of this publication that I do not believe that any one expert has all the answers. The workforce and worksites in different geographical locations have needs specific to them. Among the variables to consider are the size of local companies, type of work performed in those companies, local economy, work ethics, union involvement, employer/employee relations, and so forth.

Work hardening is not a treatment approach that will fit into the scheme of everyone's rehabilitation center. For example, if your treatment center revolves around a 50-bed hospital setting in a rural community where there is little treatment directly involving injured workers, it may not be cost-effective to open a dedicated work-hardening center. The information provided in this publication should assist you in determining how your facility can participate in meeting the needs of the injured workers in your area. If work hardening is not feasible, maybe work conditioning, which is more like traditional therapy, would better fit your center.

You will note that the generic "he" is used throughout this publication. This usage is certainly not to imply that women are never injured. The generic "he" is used in place of the "he/she" phrase, which I find to be very distracting. Within the confines of this publication, please assume that the male gender could also be the female gender in any instance.

It is my intention that this reference be readable, clear, and concise in facilitating investigation and interest in this new and exciting field. It is not meant to be a literary work of art, but rather a common sense manual that you will use again and again. The information provided is derived from years of personal experience in the field preceded by attendance in many continuing education courses provided by the pioneers of the field. This manual will not and should not replace personal attendance at conferences to learn firsthand what the experts say about work hardening. Every beginner who is providing work hardening treatment should attend educational seminars where specific problem-solving takes place with an instructor. This manual then will provide the beginner with written reinforcement of concepts learned in course work.

Feel free to copy from this manual any forms that have been developed at Milliken Physical Therapy Center (MPTC). If our forms fit your environment, it is a waste of time to reinvent them. Instead, add your logo and make them your own. You will find a list of suggested reading materials at the end of this manual. By all means, read what others have to share and integrate those concepts that appear to fit your work-injured population.

Welcome to the exciting world of work hardening in occupational/industrial rehabilitation!

ACKNOWLEDGEMENTS

This manual is dedicated to all of the people who have made its writing possible. To the contributors, thank you for taking time from your busy schedules to share your wisdom. Professionals like you encourage us to strive to make our professions better. To my business partner, Sandra M. Grant, PT, and our excellent staff, who have filled in for me to provide the time away from the office, my heartfelt gratitude. To Holly and Peggy, who provided the computer knowledge and back-up to make this manuscript a reality, thank you. And last, I dedicate this publication to my husband, who is my best friend and my staunchest supporter in all my endeavors.

CHAPTER 1

Meeting the Special Needs of the Injured Worker

THE WORK HARDENING CONCEPT

Work hardening, as a treatment approach, evolved because of the rehabilitation team's inability to meet all of the needs of injured workers. Work hardening is a multidisciplinary approach that is effective on a long-term basis. The primary goal of the specialized field of work hardening is the safe, productive return of the injured worker to the workforce. Work hardening is a structured, supervised, two- to eight-hour daily program comprised of simulated work tasks, functional activities, cardiovascular reconditioning, body mechanics, and stress management education. In this program, emphasis is placed on maximizing the individual's work capacity in order to expedite a safe, productive return to the workforce. According to the Commission on Accreditation of Rehabilitation Facilities (CARF),

> Work hardening is a highly structured, goal-oriented, individualized treatment program designed to maximize the person's ability to return to work .... Work hardening provides a transition between the initial injury management and return to work, while addressing the issues of productivity, safety, physical tolerances, and work behaviors. Work hardening programs use real or simulated work activities in a relevant work environment in conjunction with conditioning tasks. These activities are used to progressively improve the biomechanical, neuromuscular, cardiovascular/metabolic, behavioral, attitudinal, and vocational function of the person served.

Whatever definition you choose, the consensus is that this type of treatment needs to be multidisciplinary in order to be effective. With work simulation, among other activities, the injured worker also must become an active participator in the rehabilitation process.

The best way to gain a full understanding of work hardening is to compare it to traditional treatment approaches for injured workers. Work hardening is a two- to eight-hour treatment program, whereas in traditional therapy realms, the client receives a specified treatment that usually lasts about 45 to 90 minutes. With a work hardening program, the goal is to gradually increase the client's tolerance to the point at which he is functioning for a full eight-hour workday. With traditional therapy, the client returns home after his treatment and frequently spends the rest of the day completely inactive. At a time when self-esteem is usually an issue anyway, the weight gain that accompanies the inactivity may have serious psychological implications. By increasing the client's expectations of himself to eventually expect to perform in an eight-hour workday, the work hardening program assists with self-esteem issues while building physical tolerance. With more traditional therapy programs, unless the client is a very self-motivated individual, the lack of activity and resultant deconditioning may make his return to work extremely difficult and unsuccessful.

The work hardening program also attempts to re-establish adult independence and control. Ask your work-injured clients what appointments they have to keep. You may be amazed at the number of different medical professionals involved in their lives. It is easy to understand why these clients are sensing such a lack of control over their lives and their environment. This situation denies the adult client internal freedom of choice. They give up, figuring they "can't fight the system." Work hardening protocol assists the client to reclaim the adult mechanisms necessary to make good choices. This is not to say that we teach them to fight the Workers' Compensation system, but rather to work within the system while retaining their rights to self-destiny.

During the work hardening program, the client also works on self-identification of comforts and discomforts, works through feelings of frustration and anger, learns pacing, and learns how to identify what is acceptable and what is unacceptable discomfort in his life. The ultimate goal is to reacquaint the client with who he is and what is important to him. He learns that there is potential to have a good, productive life despite some discomforts. He learns to defocus on the pain and refocus on the positive aspects of his rehabilitation. Finally, he learns to take control of his body and of the connection between the mind and body.

Another difference between the work hardening program and traditional therapy is that work hardening is set up as daily therapy. The daily routine of having to "get up and go to work" can be best established by actually doing it. This statement may sound a little contradictory with making sure that the client develops independence during his work hardening program. However, the work hardening program is meant to simulate the client's job, which is a more normal part of his day-to-day routine when he is healthy. The appointments that he is assigned to keep with different medical professionals are not a part of his normal daily routine. His work routine will be a lifetime routine. The medical appointments will not. According to Maxwell Maltz, MD, FICS, author of *Psychocybernetics*,* it takes 21 consecutive days to change a behavior. By having a daily program for work-injured clients, consecutive, daily reinforcement of healthy work habits increases the likelihood that the client will be successful in establishing or re-establishing safe work practices. At our center, we frequently hear the clients remarking on how good it feels to actually be active and productive again. This also happens sometimes with clients who are reluctant to participate in the beginning. We positively reinforce participation in the program by reminding the client that this is his time set aside to facilitate healing. He is entitled to the time necessary to realize a productive return to the healthy state. It often becomes easier for clients to justify taking time out of their newly established routines at home if they can view it in this more positive light.

CLIENT DETERMINATION

Many professionals who work with injured workers have felt the frustration of reaching a dead-end in the rehabilitation process. There is the feeling that there must be something else that can be done. The client has had all of the testing available, the physical rehabilitation has proceeded as expected, and the client subjectively reports some improvement. Objectively, you, the treating professional, also find signs of improvement. However, the client is just not ready to return to the workforce. What is needed is a program to further address the physical and psychosocial needs of this injured worker. But what exactly are the special needs of this person?

---

*Powers M: Psychocybernetics. N. Hollywood, CA: Wilshire Book Co. 1960; 100.

Let's take a look at K.M.'s injury and the problems it has caused from the worker's viewpoint.

K.M. is a young, married man with two children. Four months ago he sustained a soft-tissue, low-back injury. He has undergone multiple diagnostic tests and finally was referred to physical therapy three weeks ago. He has been experiencing pain that he describes as severe enough to interfere with everything he does, and he has become fearful of attempting any increase in activity. His flexibility has diminished due to his guarded posture, and his trust in the medical profession has turned to mistrust. He says that "there just has to be something more wrong" with him. His attitude is negative and he comes across as being angry with everyone. He has gained 20 pounds. His relationship with his wife and children has deteriorated. Over the last three weeks his therapy has produced objective signs of improvement but subjectively he remains unimproved. Without even discussing the financial ramifications that add to his stress, we have the profile of a dysfunctional individual who is unknowingly working against himself in his bid to return to his former life status. Does this client sound so familiar to you that you could name him? Has he raised your frustration quotient beyond the tolerable level? By far, clients such as these are some of the most difficult to manage successfully. The frustration comes from knowing that, as a rehabilitation specialist, you can facilitate the healing process if you could just break through the barriers that the client has set up to protect himself.

The work hardening program is intended to facilitate the rehabilitation process for those clients with complicated needs including physiological and psychosocial deficits. The client described above is a perfect candidate for work hardening. The typical work hardening client has been out of work for three months or more. His cardiovascular status is compromised, and faulty body mechanics and posture contribute to ongoing biomechanical dysfunction. He exhibits a defeated attitude because of multiple failures when attempting to increase his activity level. If not angry, the client is at least skeptical when work hardening is discussed. Feasibility for employment is questionable, as issues such as timeliness, productivity, appropriate dress, safety, and social skills have not been addressed on a regular basis while the client was at home.

In summary, the work hardening client is someone who meets the following criteria:

1. Out of work three months or more
2. Compromised cardiovascular status
3. Faulty body mechanics and posture
4. Questionable feasibility for employment

5. Still experiencing pain, especially when active
6. Decreased overall body conditioning/weight gain
7. Poor physical/muscular flexibility
8. Possible psychosocial dysfunction

WHO BENEFITS FROM WORK HARDENING?

The client benefits from work hardening by building strength and endurance in a safe, supervised, structured environment. The client who truly needs work hardening will not progress well in an independent home program. The fear of increased pain, coupled with the inability to focus on any type of goal, usually sets the client up for failure. In the work hardening program, the client experiences camaraderie with fellow workers who are encountering similar problems. His safety is ensured by the presence of qualified professionals who constantly monitor his technique and assist in problem solving to enable him to complete his program daily. Small successes begin to override past feelings of failure. Social opportunities help to redevelop stagnant communication skills. Stress management classes assist the client in developing self-identification skills and assertive methods of communication. Enhanced work capabilities prepare the injured worker to re-enter the workforce at the highest level possible and with new knowledge of safe work practices.

The insurance carrier benefits as the client returns to work at pre-established safe levels. With the client's safe maximum parameters established, there is less probability that he will reinjure. Also, before the client returns to work, there is a comprehensive return-to-work plan established. All support systems are in place, which increases the chance for a successful return to the workforce.

Among the most important reasons why the physician benefits when his client is work hardened is that the client returns to work with increased awareness of safe work habits and at his maximum functional capability. Before the development of functional capacity assessments (FCAs) and work hardening, the physician was required to make an educated guess regarding safe parameters for the client's return to work. When this guess is based strictly on subjective reports from the worker, the tendency is to err on the conservative side for safety reasons. With the work hardening program, this is no longer necessary. The availability of professional input regarding his client's progress is of great value to the physician in determining the pace for return to work, i.e., light duty, half days, or combination work and continued work hardening.

The vocational/rehabilitation specialist also benefits from increased worker compliance. Pre-established safe work parameters assist this specialist in determining if the client can return to his previous employment or if a new job will be needed on a temporary or permanent basis. As part of the rehabilitation team, the vocational/ rehabilitation specialist must deal with feasibility issues as well. With improved feasibility and increased safe-work parameters gained during the work hardening process, the job market into which this worker can be placed opens considerably.

The employer gains when the employee returns to work in a timely manner. Through work hardening, the worker returns to work functioning at his optimal level. Loss of feasibility during the time the worker was out of work already has been addressed. Also, the client's work practices should safely guard him from reinjury. This is not to imply that the worker has not worked safely up until this time. However, there is a reason for this injury. Whether the injury was from a one-time trauma or a cumulative trauma, the client now must perform his job bearing in mind such issues as appropriate pacing techniques, body mechanics, "mini-breaks," etc. The employer gains value in the employee who has learned these protocols during his work hardening program.

In deciding whether or not to provide work hardening services, it is first important to recognize who benefits from work hardening. An understanding of who benefits also presents information for marketing efforts. Work hardening is a service with many benefits, but our referral sources will not deluge us with injured workers. As providers of the service, we must be prepared to educate these sources as to how work hardening is beneficial to them.

IS A WORK HARDENING PROGRAM RIGHT FOR YOUR FACILITY?

There is no formula to assure success, because there are many variables to consider. How much time and energy are you willing to devote to initiating a new service? Often, when discussing the hard work and long hours involved, potential work hardening providers are overwhelmed. Most must continue to generate income from a present source while putting in the hours necessary to search out new space, choose and order equipment, plan the new layout, and put equipment together. They also need to find time to advertise for, interview, hire, and train personnel; contract outside disciplines; and take on the many other duties involved in providing a new service. Is this something you can do right now? If so, consider the following points:

1. Am I presently treating injured workers who could benefit from this service? If so, how many?
2. Have my referral sources requested this service?
3. Would this open a new market for my facility?
4. Can my facility attract the professionals necessary to provide this service and still maintain quality?
5. What are the cost-containment issues of Workers' Compensation in my state? Will a program such as work hardening help in the cost-containment effort?
6. Is there already someone else providing this service in close proximity to my facility? If so, how will my program be different?

These are just some of the issues to consider and reviewing the "Who Benefits From Work Hardening" section may assist in making your decision. Other issues including space, equipment, and staffing will be addressed later on.

IMPAIRMENT VERSUS DISABILITY

Although impairment and disability frequently are used as interchangeable terms, they have different definitions. When working as specialists in the field of occupational rehabilitation, we have an obligation to use the proper terminology to define exactly what we are discussing. Knowing the proper terminology also provides us with an opportunity to educate others so that eventually, we all will speak the same language. The interface between the medical and industrial/workforce communities can be successful only when we understand each other's language. Let's begin by learning about impairment.

Impairment is strictly a medical determination that is made after maximum medical improvement is achieved. Of course, who decides if and when this takes place is always an area of controversy. Impairment is based on such parameters as decrease in range of motion, loss of strength, and loss of endurance. To connect any of these losses to the Workers' Compensation system, the physician first must make an association between the work and the injury or illness present.

Once the proper paperwork has been filed, the injured worker's condition is deemed nonstationary or stationary. A nonstationary determination indicates that further improvement is expected. No impairment rating is appropriate at this time. However, when the condition becomes stationary, an impairment rating may be in order. There are several physician's impairment guides from which the physician can choose to assist in making this determination. Percentages of def-

icits are given for the injured body part or for the whole body. A whole-body determination is made when there are deficits in day-to-day functions such as communication, ambulation, and the ability to feed and bathe oneself. A less tangible element to consider is pain. Because pain is not quantifiable and subjectively changes on a daily basis for some injured workers, the guides state that pain is outside the scope of their determinations. However, the guides also state that pain may be considered if the physician believes that it can be substantiated by objective clinical findings. Although the impairment rating is supposed to be objective, there is still much room for differences of opinion among physicians and therefore there are different impairment ratings based on identical information.

The determination of disability is a legal responsibility. The state Workers' Compensation board is charged with appraising disability based on the physician's impairment rating and the injured worker's ability to remain gainfully employed within a reasonable geographical area. The board looks at such factors as age, education, sex, and socioeconomic status.

The disability determination also is broken down into specific categories. This allows a disability determination to be made prior to the determination of permanent status. If a disability rating other than permanent is made, then the impairment rating will not be a consideration since it will not yet have been made. It is also possible for a worker to have an injury that causes impairment but not disability, since disability is based on the worker's ability to make a living. The following is an overview of the different, nationally accepted classifications of disability:

1. *No disability.* The worker is injured but his limitations because of the injury do not affect his job performance.
2. *Temporary partial disability.* The limitations due to the injury temporarily affect the worker's ability to do his regular job but he can perform another job for less pay. He can still work but his earning capacity is diminished for a period of time.
3. *Permanent partial disability.* The work limitations do not improve and the worker can never return to his original job. However, he can remain in the job market performing a lesser-paying job for the rest of his work life.
4. *Temporary total disability.* The injury has caused the worker to be removed from the workforce for a specified period of time with the intention of returning at some future date. He cannot earn a living at this time.
5. *Permanent total disability.* The severity of the injury prohibits the worker from ever returning to the

workforce. This decision usually is reserved for those cases in which exhaustive rehabilitation efforts have failed. At this point, the physician's permanent impairment rating as well as socioeconomic considerations are combined by the state Workers' Compensation board to determine the injured worker's future ability to earn a living. A financial settlement usually follows this determination. It is the board's responsibility to have a full understanding of the geographical area's job market in making this determination.

The issues of both impairment and disability can be very complicated. The issue of pain is considered in both cases, which muddies the waters of determination. The human emotions of anger and resentment frequently are entangled with the worker's demonstrated lack of motivation to improve. Since the worker must demonstrate an effort toward improvement, noncompliance with rehabilitation programs can become an issue. This leads to further speculation about the worker's purpose for not fully participating in the recommended treatment. Consequently, the issues of impairment and disability and exactly when these determinations should be made are not as clear-cut as they should be to make the Workers' Compensation system as fair and equitable as possible. The process of constantly re-evaluating the mechanics of the Workers' Compensation structure is a critical component in improving the quality of its results.

FEASIBILITY ISSUES

It is impossible to address a work-injured client's lack of work feasibility during conventional treatment. Feasibility issues are those qualities that make an employee valuable. They include timeliness, productivity, safety, and appropriate interpersonal skills. Timeliness involves arriving on time, arriving at all (attendance), returning from breaks on time, and remaining at the workplace for the entire day. Productivity involves quantity and quality of goods and services. Safety involves adherence to safety standards within the industry as well as those that are government regulated. Safety also relates to proper body mechanics. Appropriate interpersonal skills include the ability to interact with supervisors and fellow workers. Injured workers who develop a poor attitude regarding work in general, who do not tolerate changes within the work environment, and who aggressively respond to a supervisor's direction do not do well when returning to the workforce.

Deficiencies in any of the above areas decreases the client's chances for a successful return to work. It is not unusual to see injured workers, who at one time were excellent workers, manifest signs of work feasibility deterioration after being out of the workforce for several months. If this client has been treated at your facility or at a facility willing to share historical information regarding observed feasibility patterns, identification of the qualities that need prompt attention becomes easier. Another resource for gleaning at least a hint of possible problem areas is the FCA. If the client has been referred by a rehabilitation counselor who already knows the issues, the counselor is a great resource for this valuable information.

How Does Work Hardening Address Feasibility Problems?

Because work hardening establishes a work-like environment, immediately upon admission, the client is bombarded with the reality of a more familiar environment than the medical model he may have been exposed to during acute care treatment. Not every client will be ready for this change, so it is imperative to take the time to properly orient the new client to work hardening. We always plan to spend the first treatment day going through an orientation procedure just as if the client was a new worker beginning a new job. Think about how uncertain you were when you last began working at a new position. It is the same situation for the injured worker. The biggest difference is that the injured worker may be bringing with him considerable "baggage" depending on what course his rehabilitation has followed since his injury. If it has been smooth and cooperative, feasibility problems may be minor. However, if the course has been rough for him, you will be greatly challenged. To develop a better understanding of how to address feasibility problems through work hardening, each of them will be reviewed.

Timeliness is the most prevalent problem seen at our facility. It is easy to understand how this problem develops when the client is out of work with no schedule to keep. Initiation into the importance of timeliness begins during the orientation phase. Clients learn what is expected from them and what they can expect from our work hardening program. They are told that they must attend daily because this is their job for now. Each client punches a clock when entering the work hardening room. This provides a permanent record of attendance as well as the client's demonstrated ability to arrive on time. A schedule board is kept in the work hardening room with each client's expected arrival time. Before leaving for the day, the client is responsible for checking the board for the next day's arrival time. The client also punches the time clock for breaks and at the end of the workday. Clients' goals for timeliness may begin at a low level, such as developing the ability to remain at the work hardening center for the full assigned time. Clients at our facility are not admitted to work hardening unless they can spend a minimum of two hours with us. It is impossible to even begin to address these workers' special needs in less time than that.

With a client who has a very low physical tolerance but is otherwise very motivated, the goal initially may be to remain in an upright position and functioning for two consecutive hours. A 22-year-old woman who had been through several unsuccessful back operations really wanted to return to the workforce in some capacity. Prior to addressing her needs in work hardening, no other health care professional had helped her move toward her work goals. Timeliness and productivity were her feasibility problems. We worked on one problem at a time. Since her ability to stay at the worksite was tantamount to her work worthiness, we started with timeliness. It is important to keep the injured worker's goals in mind when dealing with feasibility issues. This young woman's goal was to return to work four hours per day. Her employer valued her capabilities and was willing to accept this time frame. It would have been self-defeating to establish higher goals that probably would have been unattainable at the time. Such a limited goal should not necessarily be accepted on a regular basis. Each case must be treated differently and evaluated on its own merit. Making a decision such as this also is much easier if you know the client from prior treatment, although an injured worker's attendance habits sometimes change when he is switched from the passive treatment mode into one of more active responsibility in work hardening.

Productivity is the ability to deliver a quality product or service at an acceptable number per unit of time, such as a factory worker producing 100 widgets every hour or a certified nurse's aide caring for six patients per day. The widgets must meet quality standards to go to market. The patients must be clean, dressed, and up in time for lunch. Productivity is the issue in both cases even though the impact is on a different population. To begin addressing the productivity issue, we may decide to direct our efforts to building strength and endurance. In a clinic setting, this would be accomplished with exercise. Exercise also may play a part in work hardening but not as the primary method. To gain strength, the nurse's aide will be given a circuit of work-related tasks to be performed over a specified period of time. These may include bathing a dummy patient, transferring the patient from bed to wheelchair, and transporting the patient to the dining room. The factory worker may be strong, but to tackle his endurance problem, he will begin some hand-sorting activities. If at his regular

job he performs his tasks standing, he also will perform the sorting tasks standing. Other skills that are reflected in productivity are the ability to follow instructions and to follow through independently to the completion of tasks. These skills are addressed with written and verbal multitask assignments specific to the client's job (Figures 1–1 and 1–2).

Safety is always of primary concern with our clients. A work environment involves the added responsibility of dealing with tools and other paraphernalia not seen in a traditional clinic. Therefore, the work hardening personnel must know the Occupational Safety and Health Administration (OSHA) rules for safety when working with these tools. At our facility, clients frequently resist wearing protective eyewear or hearing protection. They say they never wear it at their jobsite although they know that the wearing of such gear is part of the industry's guideline for safe functioning. Safe practice dictates that they must wear this gear at the work hardening facility when working with this equipment. If safety appears to be compromised by other problems such as poor vision, hearing, or sensory data intake, other health-care team members need to be involved.

On a more biomechanical level, we must assess the client's safe performance of the job task by using his body correctly. Body mechanics and posture education is initiated even before work hardening begins at MPTC. During acute care, each client attends back-care or upper-body fitness class, depending on where the injury occurred. Some clients actually need both. If the work hardening client has not attended this class prior to work hardening, he immediately is scheduled for the next available class. One-on-one training begins the first day of work hardening, and it may begin with proper posture during stretching or with immediate introduction of lifting techniques. We educate our work hardening clients based on the belief that it takes 19 to 21 consecutive days to change a habit. So, the sooner we begin to ingrain safe work postures and movements, the more likely the client is to integrate these learned behaviors on a permanent basis. The most effective method of instilling safety into the client's work tasks is to have the client demonstrate proper body mechanics during the work simulation taking place in work hardening. It thereby becomes habitual.

Interpersonal skills vary widely among the uninjured workforce so there is no reason to believe that we should not see the same in the injured population. Therefore, in the work hardening process we seek to develop acceptable behaviors. We begin the program observing the client's general attitude regarding work. If this is obviously negative, then response to fellow workers, in this case other work hardening participants, is likely to

Circuit

Occupation: Assembly Line Worker

Date	1-4	1-5	1-6	1-7	1-8	1-11	1-12	1-13	1-14
Hours	4 hrs.	4 hrs.	4 hrs.	4 hrs.	4 hrs.	6 hrs.	6 hrs.	6 hrs.	6 hrs.
Sorting (stand)	circular tiles	square tiles	red tiles	white tiles	circular tiles	square tiles	red tiles	white tiles	circular tiles
Desk Chair Lift	pivot 7#	pivot 7#	pivot 10#	pivot 10#	pivot 10#	pivot 13#	pivot 13#	pivot 15#	pivot 15#
Minnesota	1/2 tray	1 tray	1 tray	1 1/2 trays	1 1/2 trays	2 trays	2 trays	2 1/2 trays	2 1/2 trays
Push/Pull Cart	25 ft. 15#	25 ft. 20#	25 ft. 20#	30 ft. 20#	30 ft. 23#	30 ft. 23#	35 ft. 25#	35 ft. 25#	40 ft. 25#
Flip Cards						1/2 deck	1/2 deck	1 deck	1 deck
West II						level 3-5-8 10#	level 2-5-9 10#	level 3-5-8 15#	level 2-5-9 15#
Deal Cards						1/2 deck	1/2 deck	1 deck	1 deck
Bird Cage						level 2-4-6	level 3-7-9	level 2-4-6	level 3-7-9

Name_____Lucy Link_____

Figure 1–1. Independent Multi-Task Job Related Assignments

Circuit

Occupation: Plumber

Date	6-6	6-7	6-6	6-9	6-10	6-13	6-14	6-15	6-16
Hours	4 hrs.	4 hrs.	4 hrs.	4 hrs.	4 hrs.	6 hrs.	6 hrs.	6 hrs.	6 hrs.
Push/Pull Cart	sled empty	sled +10# •	sled +10#	sled +12# •	sled +12#	sled +14# •	sled +14#	sled +17# •	sled +17#
Bucket Carry	15#	15#	17# •	17#	17#	19# •	19#	22# •	22#
West IV	level 2&6 tighten 1 screw	level 2&6 1 screw	level 2&6 1 screw	level 2&6 2 screws•	level 2&6 2 screws	level 2&6 2 screws	level 2&9 2 screws•	level 2&9 2 screws	level 2&6 2 screws
Brief Tool Use (BTU)	3 screws	3 screws	4 screws•	4 screws	4 screws	5 screws•	5 screws	5 screws	5 screws
Pipe Tree	3 joints	4 joints•	4 joints	5 joints•	5 joints	5 joints	6 joints•	6 joints	6 joints

Name _____ Paul Plumber _____

Figure 1–2. Independent Multi-Task Job Related Assignments

be inappropriate. At MPTC, this client is scheduled during a slower time period in the work hardening day. Our staff provides more one-to-one interaction with the client to assist in the transition from sitting at home to taking responsibility for self and for the repercussions of inappropriate behavior. For clients demonstrating much hostility, ample education regarding appropriate venting scenarios must be provided within the confines of what is accepted behavior in work hardening. This injured worker also must participate actively in stress management sessions that are provided through the program. The client who is angry or spiteful and acting inappropriately is a difficult responsibility for one staff person. Therefore, more than one professional may need to be involved with this client.

Although all of the feasibility issues are of equal importance, I find the clients' interpersonal behavior problems to be the most challenging and exhausting. Lack of control is frequently the root cause of interpersonal skills issues. By encouraging input from the client regarding the development of his program, there is the opportunity to begin giving back some of the control he lost over his life when he became injured. The work hardening professional should begin by offering choices between two alternatives rather than leaving options wide open; this provides some guidance while at the same time offering some self-direction. Completely open-ended choices can be overwhelming for some clients.

It also is not advisable to schedule this difficult client to work on the same task with another work hardening participant at this early stage unless the other participant is very stable in interpersonal skills. It is unfair to knowingly subject an innocent party to hostility when the party may be unequipped to handle it.

After the general work hardening population acclimates to the program, however, pairing of clients with like tasks begins to prepare each of them for re-entry into the real workforce. Teamwork also can be addressed through participation in "dynohour." Dynohour is the term we have given to a dynamic activity hour dedicated to developing physical skills while enhancing the development of social skills. The clients, as a group, select one particular activity from a list. Once a week, usually for about one hour, the clients compete individually or in teams. The activities are as diverse as playing a team game such as nerf volleyball or making a fruit salad that they all share at break time. The object is to provide a selection of activities that will continue to meet the needs of clients with all types of injuries while the clients are given the opportunity to make a choice together that works for the majority.

Some examples of group dynamic hours are:

1. *Low-key Aerobics:* Have music available and plan an exercise program. Choose a person to lead the group. You also may give the clients an opportunity to plan the class themselves.
2. *Spoons:* This is a fast-moving card game that we have found very entertaining and therapeutic for the clients. (Each player is dealt four cards. Spoons (one less than the number of players) are placed on the playing surface where they can be reached. The dealer picks a card from the remaining deck. He keeps it and discards another card or passes it on. This process is continued around the table with no more than four cards in your hand at one time. The goal is to have four cards of the same set (four aces, four jacks, etc . . .) and grab a spoon. At this time, the other players grab the other spoons. The player left without a spoon gets an "S." When a player spells "SPOON," he is out. The final person left is the winner.)
3. *Volleyball/Paddleball:* Both of these games may be played either inside, sitting in chairs, or outside if you have an area available. We use a small beach ball for the volleyball, and plastic paddles with a nerf ball for the paddleball. This is a favorite activity of the clients.
4. *Fruit Salad:* We bring in many different kinds of fruit requiring various peeling and chopping techniques and the clients put together a fruit salad. They whip cream by hand and at the end of the Dynohour, we all eat the fruit salad.
5. *Ice Cream:* Bring the ingredients and a hand-crank ice cream maker and make ice cream. It is enjoyable and therapeutic at the same time.
6. *Painting Projects:* Find a large object that needs to be painted, preferably with different colors.
7. *Group Woodworking:* This is a good project to get a lot of people involved if you have people who enjoy woodworking.
8. *Latch-Hook Rug:* The yarn is cut, the pattern is drawn, and the latch hooking begins. It reinforces hand positioning and sitting or standing tolerances. Also, it initiates social interaction.
9. *Adi:* A marble game that can be competitive and challenging. You can even make a contest out of it, and the winning player can receive a trophy or certificate. (ADI is a marble game—manufactured by Worldwide Games—that starts with four marbles in each well in two rows. Pick up the marbles from one well and drop one in each consecutive well until you run out of marbles in your hand. You then pick up the marbles from the well you dropped the last marble in and repeat the process. Proceed until you land in a well without marbles, then it is your opponents turn. The object of the game is to completely empty the wells in your row. When you do this, you win.)

10. *Treasure Hunt:* Have the clients search the work area for clues. The clues should apply to body mechanics, anatomy, prevention, and so forth, to help reinforce education. For example, the clue may say "I am the poster displaying proper wrist position when lifting. Where am I?"
11. *Pictionary (Pictionary Inc.)/Trivial Pursuit (Horn Abbot Ltd.):* Games that are fun, challenging, and encourage social interaction.
12. *Videotaping:* Videotape a staff member prior to performing the planned activity, such as a series of lifts with different weights. Have the clients evaluate the tape, distinguishing correct from incorrect technique. Then tape individual clients performing the same tasks and have the group critique each other.
13. *Cloth Picture Frames:* A creative activity that involves cutting and gluing. In the end the clients have something they can bring home or give as a gift. (This is also good for a counter, or table, activity.)
14. *Cribbage/Cards:* Another fun, competitive activity. Have the winner challenge other clients or have several games going on to determine who is the winner.

Dynohour is a great time to reinforce good body mechanics, hand position, etc. With imagination and available supplies, you can come up with countless cooperative group activities.

The assigning of appropriate job tasks is the key to developing work feasibility. Therefore, a job analysis or excellent job description, or both, are necessary.

THE PHYSICAL SPACE

If your work hardening center is to be within the same building as your clinic space or somehow attached to it, a separate entrance directly into the work hardening space is strongly recommended. The primary reason for this is that the work hardening program is meant to assist the client with giving up the role of "patient" and assuming self-care and responsibility. For some clients, it is extremely difficult to give up this role. If they are walking through a clinic space where they are constantly reminded of their prior patient status, relinquishing the passive patient role becomes more difficult. One of the equipment options to consider to keep costs down and to reduce space requirements is to share cardiovascular training equipment with a clinic space. The common cardiovascular space should be between the clinic space and the work hardening space, with each entrance separate so that the work hardening client does not have to enter into the clinic space.

One of the most frequently asked questions about the work hardening physical space is "How much space do I absolutely need to begin a work hardening program?" There is no concrete answer to that question. There are many variables to consider, such as:

1. How many clients do you plan to treat at the same time?
2. What kind of equipment do you plan to have in the space?
3. Will work hardening take place in a totally separate building from traditional clinic space? If not, could your cardiovascular training equipment be shared without compromising the separateness necessary?
4. What space is available in your geographical area?
5. How many windows exist in the room?

New centers should begin with at least 1,000 square feet. This appears to be a very comfortable space to accommodate 10 to 12 clients and the equipment necessary to meet all of their needs. Of course, this will feel a little tight if all of the storage takes place within the confines of the room, but it's still quite comfortable. Storage can be built into little nooks and crannies. If 1,000 square feet sounds like too much space, look at your past growth experiences. The tendency is to look at the present needs and to outgrow the space long before the lease is up. If you are building space or purchasing space already built, you do not want to have to turn clients away, overwork your staff with huge, unmanageable, unsafe client loads, or have to add space just a few months after moving in. Because work hardening is such a new venture, it is difficult to project numbers. Nevertheless, past growth can be an accurate predictor for the growth of work hardening as the community becomes better educated to its benefits.

The physical space (Figure 1–3 through 1–9) should be open, with all areas visible to supervising staff. If your space has lots of windows, you are losing valuable wall space. It is very pleasant to have a view of the outside world, and some windows are helpful for clients who work outside and feel a bit claustrophobic without them. If you need more wall space for equipment mounting, consider building some free-standing walls. However, if they are taller than four feet high, you will lose visibility in that area of the room. Whether or not this is an issue depends upon your staffing availability.

Floor covering is always a disputed point among the experts. Concrete floor surfaces simulate many industrial settings well. However, if you work with a mixed population, there will be professionals and paraprofessionals in your program as well who work in a more office-like environment. Concrete floors also may be cold.

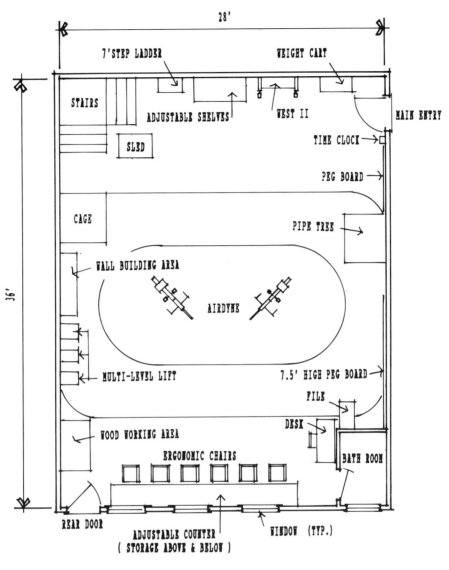

28'

7' STEP LADDER   WEIGHT CART

STAIRS

ADJUSTABLE SHELVES   WEST II   MAIN ENTRY

SLED   TIME CLOCK →

PEG BOARD →

CAGE   PIPE TREE →

WALL BUILDING AREA

36'   AIRDYNE

MULTI-LEVEL LIFT   7.5' HIGH PEG BOARD →

FILE

WOOD WORKING AREA   DESK

ERGONOMIC CHAIRS   BATH ROOM

REAR DOOR   WINDOW (TYP.)

ADJUSTABLE COUNTER
(STORAGE ABOVE & BELOW)

1008 SQ.FT.

Figure 1–3. Sample Work Hardening Layout

For most centers, a compromise—a concrete floor with indoor/outdoor carpeting—is recommended. A wooden floor with the carpeting is fine also. If your center is huge, you can have your industrial space separate from your office area. Because we did not want to run our push/pull sled across carpeting, we left a strip of floor uncarpeted and put down linoleum to prevent the runners of the sled from disintegrating on the rough cement floor.

Ceiling height should accommodate tall ladders and other equipment. A minimum of 10 feet is recommended. Ceilings higher than 10 feet may be required if you build a stair-climbing area within the confines of your primary work hardening space. We built stairs, five

on one side and four on the other, to accommodate different risers in one facility with 10-foot ceilings, and the clearance was not high enough for our taller clients.

Lighting should be adequate to prevent eye strain. There is oftentimes a fine line between adequate lighting and too much light for those clients working on the floor looking up or those at video display terminal stations. It is helpful to have lighting with individual dimmer controls to adjust to most circumstances. Free-standing, supplemental lighting may be necessary at some work stations.

Climate control that provides for the comfort for all participants contributes to the work hardening process.

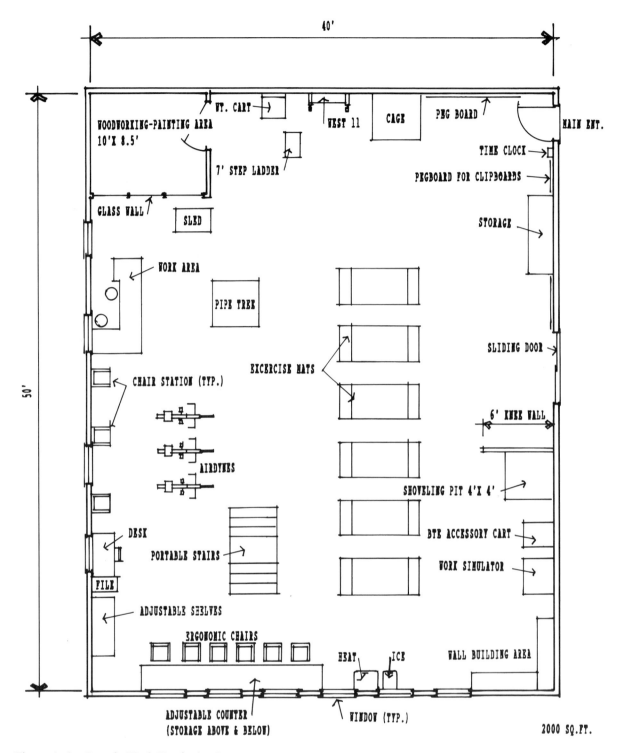

Figure 1–4. Sample Work Hardening Layout

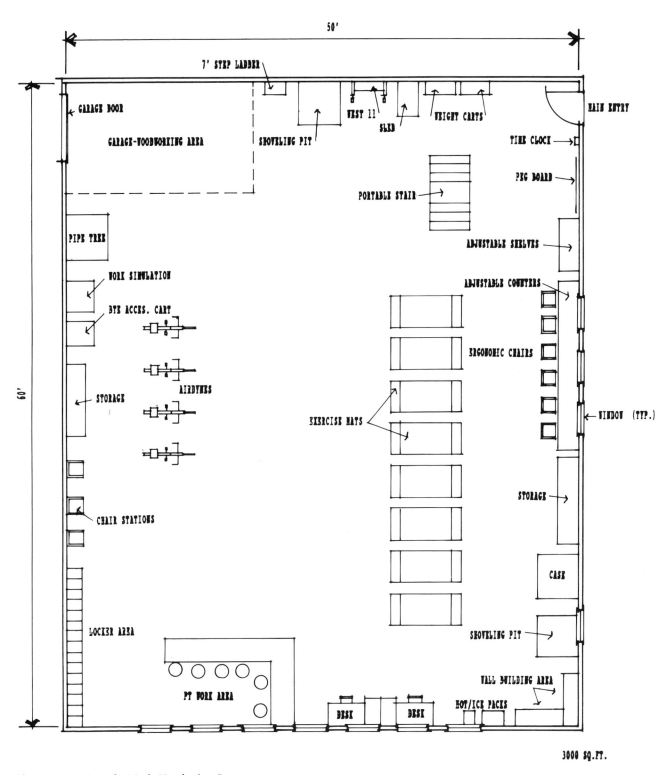

Figure 1-5. Sample Work Hardening Layout

Not all workers are fortunate enough to have ideal climate control available at their worksites, and we try to simulate work conditions as closely as possible. To be realistic, however, the definition of true working conditions, especially for those who work outside, changes with the change of seasons in many parts of the country, and these changes

(text continues on page 17)

C.O.R.E. Facility Layout

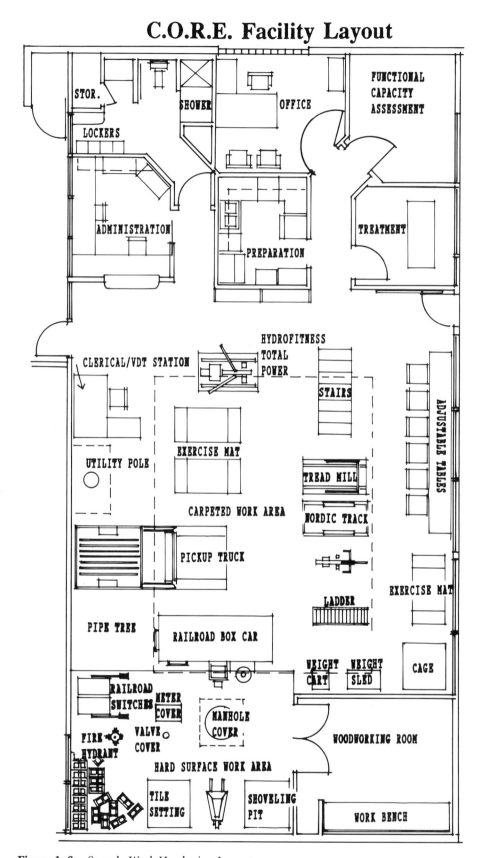

Figure 1–6.   Sample Work Hardening Layout

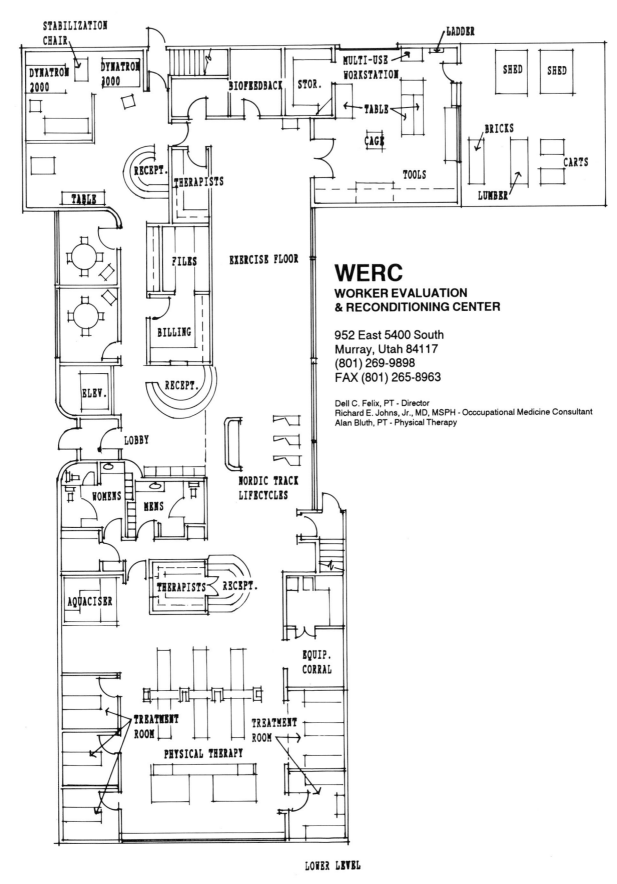

Figure 1–7. Sample Work Hardening Layout

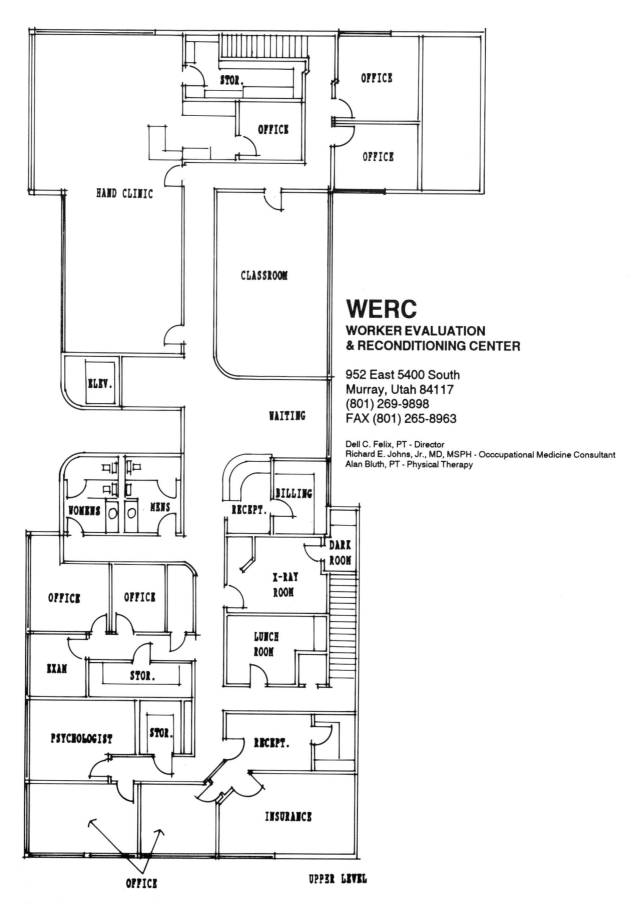

Figure 1–8. Sample Work Hardening Layout

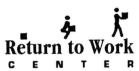

Cox Medical Center • North
1423 North Jefferson Avenue
Springfield, Missouri 65802
4 1 7 / 8 3 6 - 3 2 8 8

Bird Cage
Lifting Stations
Lift Task
Conditioning Equipment
Electrical Center
Cybex
Cybex
Gravel Pit
Warehouse
Masonry Center
Carpentry Center
Breakroom
Men's Showers
Women's Showers
Reception Department
Video Room
Exam Room
Myofascial Release
Stairs
Therapist Office
Rehab Counselor's Office
Director's Office
Medical Office Simulation
Work Simulation Equipment

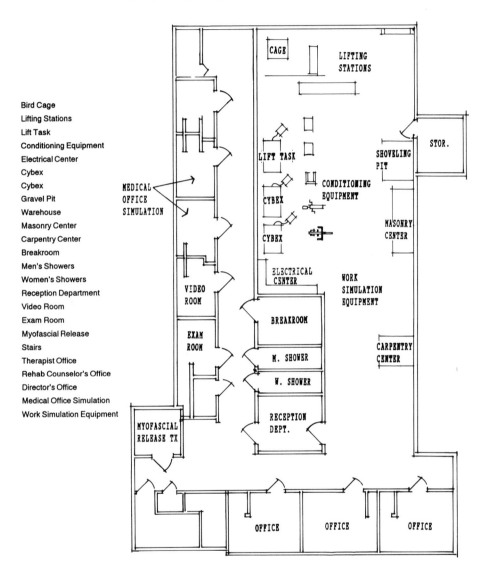

Figure 1–9. Sample Work Hardening Layout

are difficult to simulate. Work hardening participants have worked in all different climate conditions for job simulation and they generally progress better in a climate-controlled environment. Part of the workday may be supplemented with adverse climate conditions by having the clients perform part of their tasks outside.

We always have difficulty preparing injured workers to return to jobs as meat cutters or any other position involved in the meatroom where the temperatures are kept cold. The muscle contraction that involuntarily occurs because of the cold tends to cause general body tightness. Combined with the repetitive nature of meatroom work, clients tend to have a difficult time returning to this position. We have had some successes, however, even in our climate-controlled work hardening center. It is a matter of teaching layered dressing, pacing techniques, mini-break stretches, body awareness, proper body mechanics and posturing, and then having the client practice, practice, practice!

PERSONNEL REQUIREMENTS

Because safety is always the primary consideration in any environment, and is especially difficult in a group environment in which many clients must be observed at one time, the nationally accepted standard for personnel-to-client ratios is four to five clients per one work hardening professional. Each client usually can obtain the direction necessary throughout the performance of his work hardening program with this ratio. Nevertheless, there are exceptions. For example, if you have clients with perceptive problems, difficulty reading, or who need multiple cues to many of the senses in order to understand what is expected of them, that four- to five-to-one ratio should be reduced. Oftentimes, the client already has begun the program before you realize that initially he will require much more individual instruction than most clients. This is not an impossible situation in a work hardening program, especially if the client is highly motivated. But it does make it more difficult to monitor everyone for safety and technique. These clients should either be placed in a time slot during the day when the client-therapist ratio is lower or when the other clients participating are much more familiar with their programs and require less intense monitoring. The client who is having difficulty with his program was functioning adequately in the workforce prior to his injury and should be able to return to such. Frequently, the key to unlocking this client's abilities is to find which method of communication works best for him. We usually try verbal instructions, written instructions, color-coded instructions, and tactile input. We also use symbols that work for the client (Figure 1–10). In this sample • indicates a change in the program, ✓ means do these for cool down, and * means do these for warm up.

Who Performs What Functions in a Work Hardening Program?

A therapist should be the primary director in the work hardening program. I have worked in both a therapist-directed program and also in one directed by a professional in another discipline, and by far the most successful was the therapist-directed program. In the nontherapist-directed program, the primary functions of marketing/selling and the initial introduction of the program to consumers of the service and third-party payors were performed by a practitioner with a very poor understanding of what therapists do. Because she could not present the information with a full understanding of the scope of the program, it met with limited success and eventually failed. It makes sense that the successful presentation of a specialized program should be made by those who do it. This person can be either a physical therapist or an occupational therapist with industrial/occupational rehabilitation experience.

As a physical therapist, and the developer of the work hardening program at our facility, I initially had to wear many hats. Whomever assumes the director's role should recognize that, at least initially, his role will include protocol development, public relations, FCAs, insurance approvals, program writing, client orientation, and so forth. Training the rest of the staff in the philosophy desired in your work hardening center also will rest on your shoulders. After the program has been functioning for a while, and the medical and insurance communities are familiar with your program, some roles may be delegated to those in other disciplines within your facility. Initially, however, the director should be the primary person obtaining insurance approval for payment of FCAs and work hardening. This is the insurance company's opportunity to learn what it is that you do and to obtain a full understanding of what it is they are paying for. Insurance adjusters should be able to contact you directly because it is extremely difficult for secretarial personnel to answer technical questions regarding an industrial program. And, because insurance adjusters often are difficult to reach, it is best to answer all questions at the time they are asked so that insurance approval and the client's admission into the program are not delayed.

Public relations is an area that many professionals tend to shy away from, especially in the medical field. But with such a new service, it is critical that the medical community and any other disciplines involved, such as the industrial and vocational communities, have a full understanding of what work hardening is and what it has to offer. The only way to accomplish this is through public relations. We will address marketing further on.

Daily Schedule

Date	8-1	8-2	8-3	8-4	8-5	8-8	8-9	8-10	8-11
Hours	2 hrs.	2 hrs.	2 hrs.	2 hrs.	2 hrs.	2 hrs.	2 hrs.	2 hrs.	2 hrs.
Upper Body* Warm-Up	NMSS	10x	10x	10x	10x	10x	10x	10x	10x
Theraband	NMSS	10x	10x	10x	10x	10x	10x	10x	10x
Lower Body	orien-tation	stress mgmt. 45 min.	10x	10x	stress mgmt. 45 min.	10x	stress mgmt. 45 min.	10x	10x
Ergonomic Bike (Push/Pull only)	NMSS	5 min.	5 min.	7 min.•	stress mgmt. 45 min.	7 min.	7 min.	8 min.•	8 min.
Upper Extremity Exercises	NMSS	cage levels 5-6-7	Dyno. hr.	10x	cage levels 5-6-7	10x wts. added, see ex's•	cage levels 5-6-7	10x	10x
		no cage done due to heat		CA					

Name_____ Carrie Proppa _____

Figure 1–10. Sample Activities Using Symbols to Enhance the Client's Understanding

Daily Schedule

Date	8-12	8-15	8-16	8-17	8-18	8-19	8-22	8-23	8-24
Hours	4 hrs.	4 hrs.	4 hrs.	4 hrs.	4 hrs.	4 hrs.	4 hrs.	4 hrs.	4 hrs.
Upper Body* Warm-Up	10x	10x	10x	10x	10x	10x	10x	10x	10x
Theraband	10x	10x	10x	10x	10x	10x	10x	10x	10x
Lower Body Exercises	stress mgmt.	10x	stress mgmt.	10x	10x	stress mgmt.	10x	stress mgmt.	10x
Bike	stress mgmt.	10 min.	stress mgmt.	Dyno hr.	10 min.	stress mgmt.	60 min. circuit I (break)	stress mgmt.	Dyno hr. (break)
Upper Extremity Exercises	circuit I 30 min. (break)	10x (break)	circuit I 30 min. (break)	Dyno hr. (break)	15x• (break)	circuit I 30 min. (break)	bike 10 min.	circuit I 30 min. (break)	bike 10 min.
Cage	5-6-7	5-6-7	5-6-7	5-6-7	5-6-7	UE Ex. 15x	UE Ex. 15x	5-6-7	UE Ex. 15x
Circuit	upper extremity ex. 10x	45 min.	upper extremity ex. 10x	60 min.	60 min.	upper extremity ex. 15x	circuit II 60 min.	upper extremity ex. 15x	circuit I 60 min.
Body Ball Exercises	10x	10x	10x			lunch 30 min.	lunch 30 min.	10x body ball	lunch 30 min.
Lower Extremity Exercises	10x	10x	15x•	15x	15x	circuit II 60 min.	counter 30 min.	15x LE exercises	counter 30 min.
Cool Downs ✓	5x	5x	5x	5x	5x	cool down	circuit II 60 min. cool down	5x cool down	circuit I 60 min. cool down
							CA		

Name_____Carrie Proppa_____

Figure 1–10. (continued)

Besides therapists, therapist assistants and therapist aides may be involved in the direct day-to-day care of the clients in work hardening. Physical therapy and occupational therapy assistants are invaluable in the role of overseer in the work hardening program. They also can be instrumental in developing programs and helping with charting on a day-to-day basis. However, because the aide position involves on-the-job training, the aide's ability to observe proper body mechanics is frequently inadequate until the aide is thoroughly trained. If you are fortunate enough to hire someone with a health and fitness degree or have physical/occupational therapy students who do some of their clinical affiliations with you, their educational level promotes a better understanding of the nuances of proper body mechanics and therefore facilitates development of observational skills to properly supervise the work hardening client. The aide can be very helpful with such duties as copying client's programs, issuing supplies, obtaining hotpacks or coldpacks or ice massage popsicles for clients, and in physical space maintenance.

For those work hardening facilities where staff includes professionals with athletic training, or kinesiology, ergonomics, health and fitness, and related degrees, it is necessary to utilize fully their areas of expertise within well-defined parameters. Although there are preestablished, documented, acceptable parameters defining the therapist's and assistant's scope of practice, these other disciplines involved in the direct care of work hardening clients may not fall within such clearly defined parameters. Therefore, much care must go into thoroughly researching the state's legal acceptable standards. Another consideration is the third-party payor's standards for reimbursement of work hardening services.

Other professionals involved in work hardening should be vocational and rehabilitation counselors; psychologists, psychiatrists, and stress management counselors; and nutritionists and registered dieticians. As a physical therapy facility, we have contracted with an occupational therapist and a stress management specialist to provide services to our clients. Vocational and rehabilitation counseling is provided by independent agencies that are approved by the state of Maine. You will need to investigate within your state the best approach for providing rehabilitation and vocational services to your clients. We also provide two sources of nutritional counseling to our clients. One organization is a strong proponent of one particular technique and offers group counseling only. The other offers individual nutritional counseling, which is the approach our clients generally prefer. So, there are many available approaches to providing the multidisciplinary team necessary to facilitate a successful return to work for injured workers.

EQUIPMENT

There are probably as many suggestions for which equipment you should use as there are therapists with opinions. I recommend a strictly functional approach. That means avoid high-tech equipment to rehabilitate injured workers in the work hardening setting. Job simulation is the most successful technique to prepare injured workers to re-enter the workforce. Clients who demonstrate the need for a multidisciplinary approach must be able to extrapolate what is meaningful to them at the work hardening center and bring it into daily function. They cannot do that by means of a piece of sophisticated technology. If the client paints for a living, then he needs to carry ladders and paint cans, and reach, bend, and stoop while using a paint brush and roller. These are the positions and tools of his trade. He can identify with them. When he successfully climbs a ladder at the work hardening center and paints several strokes with his brush, he also learns that he can climb a ladder at home and change a burned out light bulb. Gradually, the quality of his life improves because he becomes an active participator. This is not a lesson learned without job simulation.

Figures 1–11 and 1–12 list recommended equipment to start your work hardening center and equipment you may add later. The equipment should meet your injured workers' needs generically at first, then graduate to more specifics as the client tolerates more job-specific tasks.

EQUIPMENT RECOMMENDED IMMEDIATELY

ITEM	PURPOSE	TASKS
1. Time Clock/Time Cards	• address timeliness	• punch in/out
2. Clip Boards	• promote independence	• carry daily program
3. Exercise/Instruction Sheets	• visual demo of daily tasks • written explanation • Illustrates progress • promotes independence	• use for direction of daily activities
4. Ladder	• job simulation • balance/coordination	• include in circuit • climb with receptacle • stand on 'rung' and work
5. Stairs	• job simulation • endurance	• heel cord stretches • included in circuit • climb as walk and carry
6. Bird Cage	• scapular stabilization • fine/moderate hand manipulation • body mechanics • enhance social skills	• take slats off/on • add other boards • work off ladder • multi-level manipulation
7. Multi-Level Lift Station	• job simulation • develop strength and endurance at different heights • body mechanics training	• intro to lifting • include in circuits • functional PRE's

Figure 1–11.

ITEM	PURPOSE	TASKS
8. Cement Blocks	• job simulation • body mechanics • improve cognitive functioning	• load into push/pull sled • make multi-level lift stations • use as foot rest • make pattern for block wall building • lift and carry • weight transfers • heel cord stretches
9. Pegboard	• job simulation • hand/UE manipulation • hang clipboard and supplies • scapular stabilization • body mechanics	• string art • hang items from S-hook • clothespin on pegs
10. Exercise Mats/ Pillows/Towels	• floor work	• stretching and strengthening ex.
11. Buckets	• job simulation • unilateral carry • store equipment	• painting • lift and carry • drywall
12. Crates	• job simulation • lifting receptacles • store equipment	• bilateral lift and carry • add handle to do push/pull
13. Heavy Duty Shelves	• job simulation • UE strength/endurance • body mechanics • variable height lift station • standing endurance • sitting endurance	• reaching tasks • lift and place tasks • combine with ladder to climb to lift and place • stationary standing tasks • sitting tasks
14. Multi-Level Work Stations (tables)	• job simulation • sitting/standing endurance • UE exercises • posture	stationary sit/stand tasks a. education b. hand tasks

Figure 1–11. (continued)

ITEM	PURPOSE	TASKS
15. Heavy Duty Broom	• job simulation • clients clean up after themselves • back and UE endurance • body mechanics	• sweep with and without weights on broom
16. Shovel/Pit	• job simulation • body mechanics • strength/endurance	• shovel with weights • shovel actual gravel
17. Treadmill/Track	• job simulation • cardiovascular endurance • gait evaluations • low back and LE endurance/ strength and coordination	• walking with grade and speed
18. Vacuum Cleaner	• job simulation • body mechanics • UE/Low Back endurance • cleaning	• vacuum under supervision
19. Video Equipment (Camcorder, VCR, screen , tapes)	• job analysis • postural and body mechanics education • progress record • gait analysis	• record
20. Airdyne/Ergometer	• cardiovascular training • general strength & endurance • upper body/lower body workout	• pedals and reciprocal UE • pedals only • UE only a. push/pull b. only push c. only pull
21. Push/Pull Sled	• job simulation • body mechanics • strength/endurance training	• push/pull

Figure 1–11. (continued)

ITEM	PURPOSE	TASKS
22. Push/Pull Cart with Wheels/Dolly	• job simulation • body mechanics • strength/endurance training	• push/pull
23. Dynamometers a. push/pull b. grip	a. - job analysis - measure push/pull resistance during tasks dynamic and/or static b. - assess progress grip strength	• measure push/pull resistance after loading equipment and periodically during push/pull tasks
24. Weights - Cuff, Hand-Held, Disc	• job simulation • strength/endurance training	• functional training by loading receptacles • therapeutic exercise during early stages of work hardening
25. Volumeter	• measure swelling via water displacement • feasibility/chronic pain issues	• follow directions with volumeter
26. Schedule Board	• at a glance scheduling of clients • facilitates timeliness and attendance	• therapist/assistant uses for scheduling WH, FCA's and noting doctor's appointments
27. Motivational Posters	• subliminal inspiration	• change frequently to continue having impact
28. Job Analysis Kit	• perform job analysis to better simulate job tasks during WH	• job analysis

Figure 1–11.   (continued)

ITEM	PURPOSE	TASKS
29. Slide Projector, Carousels, Screen	• Education	• Teach Back Schools, Your Healthy Upper Body, Public Relations presentations
30. General Supplies a. lumbar pillows b. anti-vibration gloves c. splints d. cervical pillows e. grippers f. tennis elbow straps g. myoflex	• facilitate postural changes and decrease environmental irritants to healing	• issue to clients PRN

Figure 1–11.   (continued)

EQUIPMENT TO BE ADDED LATER

ITEM	PURPOSE	TASKS
1. Woodworking Station a. sawhorses b. drill c. sander/sandpaper d. toolbox & tools e. level f. square g. tape measure h. saws i. staple gun j. wood burner k. wooden dowels and other wood supply l. painting equipment m. woodworking patterns	• job simulation • feasibility (safety) • self-esteem/pride • self identification • body mechanics • pacing • position tolerances	• begin by assigning small tasks, i.e. hammer 10 min., staple 10 min., drill 10 holes, hand sand one board, etc. • work up to small projects chosen by the client
2. Miscellaneous Supplies a. weaving b. straw wreath & material c. ceramic tiles d. deck of cards e. tin punching f. leather working g. electrical kits	• job simulation • self-esteem/pride • self identification • body mechanics • pacing • feasibility (production) • standing/sitting tolerances	• have the client choose a project, break it down into tasks, pace through treatment sessions to completion • good counter activities
3. Tarp	• job simulation	• used specifically for truck drivers who have to cover their loads
4. Sewing Machine	• job simulation • ADL • assess U.B./hand positions	• suggest small projects that can be broken into tasks • good counter activity

Figure 1–12.   Equipment to be Added Later

ITEM	PURPOSE	TASKS
5. Pipe Tree/Wrenches	<ul><li>job simulation</li><li>body mechanics</li><li>upper body/hand tolerances</li></ul>	<ul><li>have client assemble and disassemble using different weight wrenches and working at different heights</li></ul>
6. Sorting Rack	<ul><li>job simulation</li><li>body mechanics/posture</li><li>UE positions/tolerances</li><li>fine, moderate, and gross manipulation</li><li>social skills if multiple clients participate</li></ul>	<ul><li>client usually stands at this station sorting various materials to/from different heights</li></ul>
7. Crawford Small Parts Dexterity Test (CSPDT)	<ul><li>fine manipulation</li></ul>	Would not purchase for W.H. but could make or purchase non-standardized pieces to build hand tolerances
Minnesota Rate of Manipulation Test (MRMT)	<ul><li>moderate manipulation</li></ul>	
Bennett Hand Tool Dexterity Test (BHTDT)	<ul><li>gross manipulation</li></ul>	

Figure 1–12.   (continued)

CHAPTER 2

Choosing an Assessment System

It is necessary to obtain the client's safe functional parameters before admitting the work hardening client to the program. Choosing the method for obtaining these parameters is a highly disputed topic. The nation's leading researchers share the consensus that obtaining work parameters through the functional approach appears to deliver the most accurate results. There are many high-tech pieces of equipment that either provide for stabilized tracking of the resisted activities and/or stabilizing of the client into the machine to minimize overflow compensation from other muscle groups. What this does, however, is to take away the natural technique that the client normally uses to perform the particular task or movement and eliminates the need for the client to equally balance and coordinate a resistive activity such as lifting. These artificial methods of evaluation do not translate well into the workforce demands. As with all research and new fields, the debate will continue for quite some time. For our purposes the results of the FCA speak for themselves. We have a very successful program and have never had a client reinjured in our work center or after returning to work when using our recommended parameters.

There are certain generic qualities to look for when choosing an assessment system. One should first determine if the assessment system is truly a system or just a piece of equipment. Does it allow you to perform a total-body evaluation to obtain total-body functional parameters? If a client is referred because of a back injury, arm injury, or neck injury, it is not just this body part that returns to the workforce but also the cardiovascular system and other body musculature that have become deconditioned while the client has been out of work. It is not unusual for an injury to one part of the body to affect other parts of the body as well. If the assessment tool is a full-body evaluation system, it also will assess the client's level of participation and assist in determining the possible presence of symptom magnification syndrome, which will be discussed in Chapter 4.

Another asset to consider is the statistical data backup to the assessment system. How large is the bank from which the data is drawn? Is it a reputable, statistical group that has provided these parameters? Are the developers of the system willing to share with you, the provider, where the statistics were derived from? Is research ongoing and frequently updated? Is the population being studied generic enough to meet various facilities' needs? Are they doing any statistical studies? If so, on whom? Are there studies available concerning the noninjured population?

One of the most critical components of an assessment system, especially for a new provider of these services, is the immediate availability of assistance should a question develop during the assessment. No matter how well we are trained in a technique, there is always a tendency to feel a little less competent the first few times that we use it. A backup contact assures the accuracy of the product, in this case the results of the assessment, regardless of the experience of the evaluator. Therefore, before purchasing an assessment system, it is wise to speak with other providers using it to ascertain if the company selling the assessment system and providing the training truly is available for backup assistance in a timely manner. Unfortunately, it is very easy for the seller of the assessment system to say "you can call us anytime and we'll be glad to help." But when you need their services, no one is available to assist. This can be a very unnerving experience if you happen to be in the middle of an assessment and the client does something that you have never seen before. Your goal, as the assessor, is to make sure that you do not do anything that affects the validity of the outcome of the assessment. The "fake it till you make it" mentality does not apply here.

Also consider if the assessment system is reliable. In other words, on repeated trials, do the same patterns develop? During an assessment, the assessor should never expect specific numbers. However, the assessor should be looking for some type of pattern to develop within the different areas evaluated. For instance, if we are measuring grip strengths using a JAMAR dynamometer (Preston) we know that on repeated trials in the different grip widths, we should obtain a bell-shaped curve on a normal, uninjured hand. This is a pattern that we expect based on prior research and statistics. The assessment system used should provide expected, acceptable patterns for the activities performed throughout the assessment.

As evaluators educated in biomechanics, each assessment specialist brings with him a baseline body of knowledge regarding expected patterns of behavior. We already use these patterns when evaluating in our clinical practices. When, for instance, we have the client perform a straight leg raise in a supine position and then have the client perform knee flexion to extension in a seated position, we have expectations of observing the same degree of hamstring flexibility with the same behaviors and complaints of pain. If the expected pattern does not develop, we question the client's subjective reporting reliability. The assessment system protocols should be thorough enough to make some of the same types of determinations with a high degree of confidence based on prior studies.

Cost-effectiveness of providing the service of FCAs is a critical component to consider when choosing an assessment system. If it takes you six hours, for example, to perform the evaluation and another two hours to put the evaluation together and dictate it and then another 30 minutes to edit the report received from your typist, it is going to be very difficult for you to obtain appropriate reimbursement for your services. Most Workers' Compensation systems, whether they are state-run or independent insurance carriers, could not bear the cost of a lengthy FCA such as this. Therefore, a system for evaluating a client for beginning functional capabilities for a work hardening program, or for a client who may be returning to the workforce immediately, must provide reliable, valid, safe parameters in a timely manner. If the assessment fits reasonable time frames but has not proven to provide safe results, it is a useless system.

One of the best methods to determine if the assessment system has been accurate in providing safe parameters is to ask whether there have been any follow-up reinjury studies after the clients' return to the workforce. If so, ask for at least an abstract regarding the results of the follow-up study. If not, question claims of the success of this assessment method in safely returning injured workers to the workforce. It would be unrealistic to think that every client that you return to the workforce always will remain injury-free. There are too many variables that are not within our control to make this guarantee. Nevertheless, every effort must be made to accurately determine safe functional parameters prior to returning an individual to the workforce.

Even if the primary purpose of the FCA is to determine return-to-work parameters, suggestions about correcting observed deficiencies, such as poor, unsafe body mechanics, can be provided along with the worker's demonstrated safe work parameters. Safety of the injured worker is always the primary consideration. We cannot make the referring party follow the recommendations, but we can inform them when their employee's safety is in doubt for any reason. It is then up to the employer to follow-through on recommendations to assure the worker's safety on the job.

During an FCA, no body mechanics education nor any joint-specific musculoskeletal evaluation should take place. This is again based on the fact that it takes 21 consecutive days to change a behavior. If a change in body mechanics is attempted during the assessment, and this attempt results in changes in the demonstrated functional parameters of the client, then we have not truly obtained the client's functional capability. When that client returns to the workforce, he will perform his work tasks with the same techniques he always has used, not with techniques we forced him to use during the FCA. If we attempt to change body mechanics during the FCA, we could be compromising the worker's future safety because of inaccurate information. We can work on changing them later when the client is afforded the time needed to do so.

There are many assessment systems from which to choose. It is not an easy choice to make. A careful study of what each system has to offer is pertinent. Some facilities, especially in Canada, already have a large client population committed to them before their work hardening centers even open. These facilities have chosen to develop their own assessment systems. This is acceptable as long as the person who develops the system is someone with considerable experience in this area. If not, then many years will follow before the assessment system developed is truly a credible system. Standardization of both equipment and format is crucial to the development of a reliable, valid assessment system. The FCA area of study is exciting and constantly evolving. Ongoing research, revamping of established assessment systems and protocols, and the development of new systems offer many choices to the professional community providing this valuable service.

WHY DO I NEED AN FCA?

Prior to the development of FCAs, the usual approach to determining an injured worker's return-to-work status was to ask him what he could do. The physician was forced to make an educated guess and fill out the physical-functioning form requested by the employer. This potluck system frequently resulted in return-to-work parameters that were very conservative and prevented the injured worker from returning to his previous job—or even worse, from returning at all—since there would be nothing available at his worksite within these low functional parameters. It was obvious that a more systematic approach was needed. With the advent of work hardening, it quickly became apparent that initial safe parameters were necessary. Before beginning a client in a work hardening program, it is imperative to establish safe levels of function as guidelines with which to build and improve the client's physical and psychological functioning. The FCA provides information regarding:

1. Whether the client has other needs before or instead of work hardening.
2. Workday tolerances.
3. Resistance tolerances.
4. Position tolerances.
5. Cardiovascular condition.
6. General worker attitude.
7. Validity of participation (whether or not the client fully participated in the evaluation or tried to manipulate the results).

There are also other types of functional assessments that provide more specialized information. For example, KEY Functional Assessments, Inc., produces a cardiac assessment specifically designed for the cardiac client who is returning to the workforce. As the Americans with Disability Act (ADA) was signed into law July 26, 1990, by President Bush, consideration also should be given to performing job placement assessments. Job placement assessments provide specific information regarding a potential worker's capability to perform the job tasks required of that particular job position. The ADA stipulates that "Employers may devise physical tests and other job criteria and tests as long as the criteria and tests are job-related and consistent with business necessity. For example, an employer can adopt the physical criterion that an applicant be able to lift 50 pounds if that ability is necessary to an individual's ability to perform the essential functions of the job in question."* This law makes job placement assessments an excellent tool by which a business can determine work parameters for its job applicants. However, job placement assessment would never be performed on a client with a fresh injury. A full body FCA is absolutely necessary before returning this client to the workforce.

---

*Golden M: The Americans of Disability Act of 1990. J Voc Rehabil 1991; 1(2):14.

SPECIALIST SURVEY

To provide an eclectic overview of current FCA methods, philosophies, and development, several leading specialists were questioned. Their written replies are as follows:

Q As a provider of work hardening, do you use an FCA to determine entrance parameters?

Brenda G. Allen, PT—Assessment Centers Technology (ACT), 2501 N. Glebe Road, Suite 100, Arlington, VA 22207; Tel: (703) 527-9355

A Yes. We do require that each client undergo an FCA to determine baseline information, as well as to determine whether or not the client is an appropriate candidate for a work hardening program. We have developed our own system, which has both new methods and incorporates methods previously described and supported in the literature.

To establish the client's full participation or lack thereof, we incorporate information gathered by the examiner during the most obvious means of determining maximum effort. For example, in some cases, when specifically asked to perform a deep squat, some clients claim that they cannot perform the activity. But when, in the functional portion of the evaluation, the client is asked to lift a box from floor level, he performs the activity without difficulty. This is only one simple example of how the examiner's observation skills are imperative in identifying submaximal effort.

Dr. Matheson has researched thoroughly and published his findings using the JAMAR Hand Dynamometer as an indicator of a client's level of effort. His software package, which graphs the results, is a great means of explanation to referral sources.

The WEST Tool Sort is another helpful method that is on the market. This activity looks at the client's thought process when he is asked about performing various functional tasks. It does not necessarily indicate full participation, but it can clue the examiner in on whether the client perceives his "disability" consistently with the amount of effort that he demonstrated during the evaluation.

The two above-mentioned established systems are helpful in terms of having a standardized and objective means of looking at maximal effort and the client's perception of his disability. By combining several of these types of processes, we move toward objective evidence on which to base functional decisions. However, none of these systems can stand alone. The examiner must be trained in how to use these types of methods and how to interpret the data.

With the economic status of the U.S. today, everyone is interested in the almighty dollar. In our program at ACT we encourage referral sources to get the clients to us as soon as the treating physician determines medical stability. This facilitates a timely return to work for the injured worker, a successful case for the doctor, and the most cost-effective treatment plan for the insurance company. The longer the case lingers on, the more difficult case resolution becomes.

Also, not only does Assessment Centers Technology (ACT) provide functional capacity evaluations and a work hardening program, but we also provide job task analyses and worksite redesign. By combining these services, we can determine clearly whether the client can or cannot meet the physical demands of a specific job. And, if he or she cannot, we can make recommendations of how the employer may modify the job to accommodate the needs of the client and prevent recurrence of injury.

John Deblasis, MS, PT, ATC—Physical Therapy Services, 137 Waddles Run Road, Wheeling, WV 26003; Tel: (304) 242-5080

A The FCA that we use is a combination of Blankenship and Matheson. We have added isometric strength tests established by Keyserling as well. The FCA is preceded by clinical evaluation of the client's major complaint. Inconsistencies are ascertained from both parts of the evaluation process.

The benefits that we perceive include the following:

1. The client receives needed education on posture and mechanics.
2. There is an opportunity for the client to determine his or her ability to return to work in a controlled environment.
3. We can provide the client with a strong home exercise program for prevention.

Michael R. Noonan, PT—CORE, Center For Occupational Rehabilitation & Education, 5232 E. Pima Street, Suite D, Tucson, AZ 85712; Tel: (602) 327-1159

A We use the Key Functional Capacity Assessment to determine entrance parameters. Weaknesses that we see are as follows:

The client is questioned about sitting tolerance while sitting tolerance is being assessed. Standing tolerance is assessed at the end of the activities and the client often has a complaint of being fatigued from the rest of the exam and this may interfere with his true standing tolerance. Also, when determining weights achieved, there is quite a bit of repetition to get up to the maximum weight, so not only strength but fatigue plays a factor because of the number of repetitions and the lack of rest between repetitions. This may alter what a client actually can do—one repetition maximum. The price in training an assessor also can be viewed as a weakness to our business manager.

The strengths of the Key FCA are as follows: The computer program facilitates timeliness and punctuality in an organized, easy-to-read report. Because patients determine their own end points they can be directly responsible for what they achieve. In litigation this is advantageous and it also builds safety into the exam. Another advantage is that the Key FCA tests functional activities in functional planes of motion rather than single plane movement, which is not used in everyday life. Probably the best advantage is that the validity determination is very good secondary to the analysis of six components separately and with each other.

Dell C. Felix, PT—Worker Evaluation & Reconditioning Center (WERC), 952 East 5400 South, Murray, Utah 84117; Tel: (801) 269-9898

A I do use an FCA prior to a client's entrance into a work hardening program. I do not use any specific established system. I have combined several ideas that I have seen in the past from Matheson's group to some of Blankenship's. Basically, I respond to the needs of those who have asked questions of me in the functional capacity of the individual.

Q Do you find FCAs useful as tools for returning injured workers to work with more accurate work tolerance and/or sooner than without them?

Michael R. Noonan, PT

A What I see as a special benefit to providing work hardening to my clients is giving them sort of a "resume" concerning their physical demands from which they can seek work. Also, we address pain management techniques with our stress-management program as well as daily work hardening program. I feel we provide a nonthreatening environment to activate, motivate, and educate our clients.

Dell C. Felix, PT

A I basically see our work hardening as an end point to their rehabilitation and work injuries. I see it as a means by which individuals are able to demonstrate control of symptoms, increased tolerances, and increased confidence in returning to the workplace.

The basic parameters I look for in beginning a work hardening program are:

1. Some control of symptoms.
2. A clear desire on the client's part to improve and return to an active life-style.
3. A need to improve body mechanics, overall strength, endurance, and work tolerances. A full participation in maximum voluntary tests also is helpful.

We are adjacent to a sports mall that allows us to emphasize the physical conditioning aspect of work hardening. We provide class work each week in nutrition, stress management, body mechanics, exercise physiology, and coping with injuries. We have indoor and outdoor work simulation areas.

Annette Evans, OTR—Return to Work Center, Cox Medical Center North, 1423 North Jefferson Avenue, Springfield, MI 65802; Tel: (417) 836-3288

A An FCA is used for all new clients. Over the years, we have developed our own system, which includes an initial interview and history, work task ability, upper-extremity and lower-extremity and trunk-musculoskeletal evaluation, and psychosocial assessment. The guidelines used to establish a client's full participation are placed throughout the evaluation. Dynamometer curvatures, reported versus observation of actual abilities, Cybex back evaluation results, straight-leg raise, axial loading, and simulated rotation are some we use.

Of the established systems that we use, it is this therapist's opinion that all have inherent weaknesses, as there is not enough evidence of viability for any of the above methods to conclude that various responses to procedures indicate a lack of participation or rather client's motive for this lack of participation. Many variables must be considered, such as pain, fear, fatigue, lack of full understanding of instructions, or merely individual characteristics of behavior. Thus, the optimum guideline would be to document carefully objective and subjective data obtained from a variety of methods to present an overall picture of the client's effort and participation.

Timothy J. Bayruns, PT—Cherry Hill Physical Therapy; Work Capacity Assessments, P.A., Kingsway Medical Center, Suite 7, 207 South Kings Highway, Cherry Hill, NJ 08034; Tel: (609) 795-9515

A As a part of work hardening services I do use a functional capacity system, primarily the Key FCA system. Knowing that things seldom function in a vacuum, I also have attended Blankenship's seminars and Matheson's seminar, as well as Karen Johnson Schultz's seminar on Upper-Extremity Capacity Assessment. I feel that in general some of the established systems lack flexibility in their approach to the evaluation. I believe that having a well-rounded experience in the entire work hardening assessment philosophy goes a long way in helping fill those blanks. I would encourage any new therapist just entering this field of physical therapy/occupational therapy, to gain experience through attending as many seminars as possible to get a well-rounded viewpoint.

Q As a rehabilitation/vocational counselor, do you find FCAs useful as tools for returning injured workers to work with more accurate work tolerances and/or sooner than without them?

Jane Gerrish—Crawford Health and Rehabilitation, 95 High Street, Portland, ME 04101; Tel: (207) 871-7236

A FCA's are useful to more accurately define work tolerances. They can produce those sooner in some cases, especially if the physician(s) will not provide a work capacity. I do need to add that for purposes of working within the Maine rehabilitation system, a statement of functional capacity is needed from the treating physician, for use by the rehabilitation provider (as compared to one obtained through a second opinion for example). So, if one is obtained by a source other than the treating physician, review and approval by that physician would be needed to use that statement of functional capacity. Overall, these assessments are far more comprehensive than statements given by many physicians, when especially "light" duty is the recommendation, and more accurate in measuring effort. The validity report is also valuable in assessing rehabilitation outcome.

I see my role as that of facilitator and advocate/educator. I facilitate communication, as needed, among all involved parties—attorney, treatment providers, injured worker, employer of injured worker, and potential employers. My role also involves speaking for the worker, where indicated. Interwoven with this function is educating all involved regarding the rehabilitation system, its processes, and my role in relation to those processes.

Q Please explain the development and philosophy of your FCA.

Margot Miller, PT—The Polinsky Advantage, 530 East Second Street, Duluth, MN 55805; Tel: 1-800-FCA-5083

A The Polinsky Functional Capacities Assessment was developed at The Polinsky Medical Rehabilitation Center in 1981 in response to our physicians' need to have more specific and accurate information regarding a patient's ability to do work. As seen traditionally, it was the physicians' responsibility to indicate a worker's readiness to return to work as well as to identify the level of return to work. Without having specific and objective data, the medical releases they provided were often subjective and general in orientation. Therefore, in an effort to identify objectively and accurately a worker's physical abilities and to ensure a safe return to the workplace, a functional test was developed.

After an extensive literature search and reviewing the various quantification methods available including isometric testing, isokinetic testing, manual materials handling testing, etc., our basic premise was that a dynamic, functional evaluation was needed. Our original FCA involved testing 17 activities—lifting, carrying, bending, reaching, and so forth. From the beginning, the following assumptions were deemed critical to our approach:

1. *Two-day testing.* The Polinsky FCA is a five-hour assessment performed over a two-day format. This allows the therapist to observe and document the effect day-one testing has on the worker. All weighted activities are repeated on day two. Worker reliability and consistency are examined more closely in a two-day approach.

2. *Physical and occupational therapists.* Physical therapists and occupational therapists have a strong background in muscle function and body movement and thus the expertise to "test" function. All therapists performing the Polinsky FCA are required to attend a two-day educational session prior to performing FCAs. The FCA focuses on the clinical skills and knowledge of the therapist.

3. *Safety.* The philosophy of the FCA is that it is critical for the therapist to provide education regarding proper body mechanics to the worker being evaluated. Poor body mechanics or unsafe body movements make injury more likely. A referrer is assured that the weight loads listed on an FCA report are safe maximum loads, and furthermore the worker is capable of safely returning to work at that level.

4. *Standardization.* Tester bias and subjectivity are eliminated with standardized testing format. The activities tested during an FCA utilize standard body positions. The testing protocol is reviewed thoroughly during the educational training session and a detailed procedure manual goes to each facility purchasing the FCA.

5. *Comprehensiveness.* The FCA tests body performance during a variety of activities. Both abilities

and limitations are documented as well as reasons for limitations. All major muscle groups and joints are stressed a number of times in a variety of positions, giving a more complete picture of the worker's overall physical ability. Strength, endurance, pace, repetitions, and coordination all factor into the picture. Cardiovascular status is critical as well when determining worker readiness to return to work. The comprehensiveness of the FCA leads to appropriate placement of the worker at the worksite to avoid further injury.

6. *Objectivity.* To effect a safe return to the workplace, test data must be based on observable and measurable phenomena. Therapists administering the FCA realize the importance of careful observation and documentation. In addition, all the test activities have specific parameters and requirements outlined in detail for the therapist. The FCA becomes a performance indicator when objectivity is the rule.

7. *FCA Network.* By far, the most distinguishing feature of our assessment is the FCA Network Concept. Polinsky is committed to supporting providers of the FCA in a variety of ways: clinical expertise and consultation, legal consultation, national marketing, research and data collection, and continuing education seminars, to name a few. Polinsky leads the way in developing not just a superior evaluation, but a whole network of services and information resources.

Over the last several months we have made some enhancements to our original FCA, beginning with a name change. We are now the Polinsky Advantage. An overhead lift and unilateral carry were added to the testing protocol, making for 20 activities tested over the two days. A computer software program was written specifically to generate the FCA report, and it has proven to be a cost-saving and time-saving measure for our providers! Lastly, having an 800 phone number makes the Network even more readily available to all our providers. Our providers know that our support is their advantage!

The Polinsky FCA testing format combines a thorough musculoskeletal examination followed by the assessment of 20 functional activities. Objective findings such as strength, endurance, pace, repetitions, related limiting factors, etc., are documented. After completion of the FCA, a report summarizing the findings is written. The FCA report has been praised consistently by physicians, attorneys, and industry for its objectivity and clarity. (See FCA Summary Letter in Appendix section.)

Since the first FCA was given, client performance data has been collected and analyzed. The Data Bank was established to:

1. Provide a means to look at "average" performance for injured clients.
2. Establish correlations between performance on functional activities that are alike or use similar body positions or muscle groups, and/or between functional activities and gender, age, and injury.
3. Establish factors that will indicate a successful return to work.
4. Establish data that will indicate when a client has fallen outside one or two standard deviations to indicate the need for a closer examination of performance, consistency, and motivation.
5. Provide information regarding FCA activity throughout the FCA Network.

Another kind of data available to Polinsky providers is a Normative Data Bank. This data has been extremely useful in comparing the injured client performance to his or her normal, uninjured counter-part. The normal data is also useful when establishing rehabilitation goals for the injured client.

In the area of work hardening, the FCA's first use will be to document whether work hardening is necessary by comparing the client's abilities and limitations to the job demands. The FCA thus provides the basis of and framework for a work hardening program.

Polinsky's philosophy and definition of work hardening is that it is a multidisciplinary team approach to facilitate the return of an injured worker to maximum function. Work hardening is therefore the process of getting the worker physically and psychologically ready for work. Recommended disciplines include physical therapy, occupational therapy, and psychology. The three major components of the actual program are physical restoration (exercise), job simulation, and education and support groups. The Polinsky approach of returning injured workers to work is well tested, practical, and easily implemented at a reasonable cost.

CHAPTER 3

Rehabilitation Barriers

SYMPTOM MAGNIFICATION SYNDROME

Leonard N. Matheson, Ph.D., of the Employment Rehabilitation Institute of California, having worked with injured workers over many years, observed that many injured workers are inappropriately labeled "malingerer," with all of the negative connotations that the word implies. Matheson believes that, as professionals working with the injured population, we have a responsibility to not only look at the client's behavior but also to try to separate the behavior observed from the motivation for that behavior. If we can do this, the injured worker may be treated more appropriately and the chances for a successful course of rehabilitation may increase.

According to Matheson, there are three types of what he terms "symptom magnifiers." The Type 1 symptom magnifier is called the "refugee." This person perceives himself as an irreplaceable part of the community and family. He feels that there is nobody out there who can take over his responsibilities, so he plods along without seeking outside assistance. In his case, the symptoms provide an escape from this unresolvable conflict.

The Type 2 symptom magnifier is the "game player." This is the person usually labeled malingerer. He is an opportunist who sees his symptoms as a way to procure something he has wanted. This oftentimes is a financial settlement, but not always. The game player is usually someone with a history of robust goals but poor goal attainment.

The Type 3 symptom magnifier is called the "identified patient." This person has lost all other roles in his life except that of being a patient. Everything he exists for revolves around this role. He is unable to be a spouse, parent, friend, or worker. Any attempts at conversation usually result in frustration for the listener because every topic always comes back to this person's patient role.

Our work hardening center has been successful in returning Type 1 and 2 symptom magnifiers to the workforce, but the Type 3 symptom magnifier really needs individual, intense counseling before we can help. Against our better judgment, we have twice admitted clients to work hardening, on a trial basis, whom we thought were "identified patients." The physicians insisted that work hardening was the best method to deal with these individuals. In both cases, within two weeks, suffering through dreadful behavioral difficulties, the clients were discharged because they were inappropriate for this setting. Since these experiences, our center has not been pressured into admitting anyone who demonstrates signs of Type 3 symptom magnification. The object of work hardening is the successful return of clients to the workforce. We want to facilitate successes in their lives, not add to the list of failures. I almost can guarantee a failure with the "identified patient" in a work hardening environment. These clients must learn to deal successfully with their psychological well-being before moving on with their physical well-being.

OTHER REHABILITATION BARRIERS

There are many barriers to rehabilitation other than symptom magnification. During the many years that I have been providing work hardening treatment, I would like to think that I have seen it all! Nonetheless, I am sure that I have not. Every day is a learning experience in human behavior. I find that I must constantly call upon not only my professional experience and expertise but also upon my life experiences. It is sometimes difficult for the less life-experienced staff to respond spontaneously to a client's unusual behavior. If you find this situation at your facility, plan to conduct spontaneous team problem solving, pooling all of your experience. In addition, regularly scheduled team meetings should provide multidisciplinary expertise to facilitate smooth operation in the work hardening center. It seems as though the more experienced we become, the fewer overwhelming problems develop. It becomes easier to extrapolate the solutions from prior similar experiences. The work hardening staff also recognizes potential problem areas earlier on. A more concrete discussion of specific barriers observed at our facility may assist in problem solving at your facility. If you are already working in a seasoned facility, you probably could add to the list.

Pacing problems are observed in a small percentage of our work hardening population. Working too fast or too slow is a barrier that affects feasibility—mainly safety or productivity, or both. The staff begins pacing with daily verbal reminders provided to the client. However, the clients must learn to track their work pace independently with a set productivity goal established beforehand. A metronome works well for repetitious tasks. Hourglass or mechanical egg timers are also helpful with pacing. Other methods include checking off each activity as it is accomplished and documenting the number of times the task was completed within a specific time period or documenting starting and ending times for each activity.

Identification as to the reason a client has pacing problems is helpful but not always possible. Clients who work too slowly usually are influenced more easily than those who work too fast. Oftentimes, the slow movers function that way because of discomfort. As they work through the pain control techniques available to them, increased speed becomes natural without a loss in quality of the tasks accomplished. For the slow worker, a minimum number of tasks per unit of time is set.

The problem clients are the "spitfires" who have zipped around all their lives in everything they do. They were injured partially because their bodies did not respond positively to the demands placed upon them. They equate slowing down with wasting time. Relaxation techniques are helpful in dealing with the stress they feel when instructed to slow down. Of course, stress management is provided to all clients in work hardening. But these clients need constant reinforcement of the techniques or they do not improve their pacing problem. For the fast worker, a maximum number of tasks is allowed per unit of time. This technique does not create competitiveness or embarrassment because the client is only working to improve his record against his previous record. The other work hardening participants do not know each other's goals unless they choose to share them.

Family issues can be some of the most difficult to address. Family members who are unsupportive of the client's rehabilitation can sabotage the clients' efforts. It would appear that supporting a spouse would be natural to promote a return to a more healthy life-style. Nevertheless, family members each have their own agendas to which we have no access. For example, Bob has had a back injury for six months. He subjectively reports some improvement but not enough to allow him to return to his job. His wife has tried to be supportive throughout the rehabilitation process. She has had times when she just could not listen to one more complaint and was glad she worked outside the home to get

away from him. But now, at last, his complaints are under control. When he begins work hardening, he again complains constantly while at home. His complaints while in work hardening are expected and appropriate and are resolved with some degree of success. But his wife only knows what she sees and hears at home. She quickly tires of the complaints and asks him why he doesn't stop his program if he is so much worse. The seed is planted or, if it was already there, it becomes supported and legitimized. This is a scenario for failure. Without the wife's support the client drops out of the program. The wife's remark was innocent but was just what the client needed for an excuse to drop out.

One of the best methods for dealing with lack of information regarding the work hardening program is to include the non-injured spouse. We invite spouses to make an appointment to visit the facility and ask questions and observe what their mate is doing. We stress the important supportive role each spouse can play. The unknown can be an enemy to successful rehabilitation.

The other extreme is the overbearing spouse. The overbearing spouse frequently will attend work hardening along with the client, whether he or she is invited or not. The spouse openly criticizes everything the client does, makes negative comments to the therapists and other work hardening participants, writes in red pen on the client's program to make sure the therapist sees it, and generally demoralizes the atmosphere. Perhaps these particular work-injured clients continue to attend work hardening because it is one of the few aspects of their lives over which they feel they have any control or success. The other possibility is that it removes them from the home environment, where more severe criticism abounds. In this situation, one successful approach begins with a long, private discussion with the overbearing spouse. First, the therapist should try to obtain some sense of motivation for this behavior. Frequently the spouse will not overtly share this, although feelings of anger and frustration surface as predominant reasons. If the therapist can gain the spouse's trust, he may point out that this time that their spouse is spending in work hardening might be a good time to take care of some of their own needs that have been neglected during the intense care required by the injured spouse. Months of caring for an injured spouse can manifest in anger when the healthy mate always "takes a back seat." If the overbearing spouse's behavior continues, then the only alternative is not to permit the noninjured spouse to attend. Depending on the power of the dominant figure, you also could lose the client.

If there are dependent children in the family, acting out behavior also may enter the picture. Those who have children know how sensitive they are to changes in the household routine. The added pressures inherent to the situation of an out-of-work, injured parent render an immediate change within the home situation. Since children do not know how to handle these changes that also affect them, they alter their behavior to get their needs met. Since the parents' roles dictate that the child's needs come first, it is confusing for the child to see a parent's needs coming first, especially over a protracted time period. Depending on the severity of the situation, this may be necessary for a while. Work hardening clients have a difficult time justifying time for themselves when a child is pouring out negative energy to gain attention. Some of our clients restructure their whole lives to address this worry positively. Even if the client can manage to take care of the child's behavior difficulty, it is an ever-present distraction on a subconscious level. This is energy-draining for the client and clearly can interfere with the rehabilitation process.

Financial difficulties are oftentimes at the root of a client's lack of progress. Clients cannot think about injury rehabilitation if their basic resources are in jeopardy. Functioning on two-thirds of their income as provided under Workers' Compensation law or on no income if the case is being controverted and they are awaiting a hearing, is stressful. Clients have been evicted from their apartments or have had their houses repossessed by the banks because they could not meet their mortgage payments. Their health care insurance is dropped by the employer or they have to choose between eating and paying for health care coverage. Usually, the basic needs to feed, clothe, and shelter the family come first. Understandably, the problem of not enough income to make ends meet infiltrates the client's every waking thought. Negative behavior and resentment at being in this position make rehabilitation very difficult. The very real fear of losing the creature comforts that have taken a lifetime to gain and of being reduced to struggling to care for the basic needs of life can be overwhelming.

Lack of education becomes a serious detriment to rehabilitation when it interferes with the client's ability to understand the exercise and body mechanics techniques. These concepts include proper stretching without injuring, body mechanics, daily participation, work habits training, therapeutic exercise techniques, and cardiovascular monitoring during rehabilitation. The uneducated client or the client with perceptual difficulties presents a danger to both himself and those around him because he may confuse written instructions or pictures. Oftentimes, this client will be jovial and try to laugh off the entire rehabilitation process to cover up for his feelings of inadequacy. Monitoring this client takes a perceptive professional with excellent communication skills. Early detection permits the client to avoid embarrassment and to try other techniques to learn the necessary information. The therapist must present different learning approaches to detect the learning style that fits the client. The client with these difficulties requires much more one-to-one time than usual. Scheduling the client in a time slot where this assistance can be provided is crucial to his success.

The client with a learning difficulty or who cannot read also presents difficulty in returning to the job market, especially if he was a hard laborer and will not be able to return to this type of work due to the severity of his injury. The barriers to returning to the workforce are, first, that the client is not educationally equipped to acquire new skills that fit within his physical capabilities, and second, the geographical area in which he lives may offer predominantly heavy labor work. The client may have an excellent work ethic but cannot return safely to the workforce where he lives. This client may indeed be unemployable. A course of work hardening may increase his physical capabilities, but may not be enough to assist his re-entry to work in his geographical area.

Alcohol and drug abuse are grounds for discharge from a work hardening program. At MPTC, we make every attempt to direct clients with a problem to available assistance in the area. We always inform the physician when we suspect a problem and try to get him involved. We also are very direct with the client. The safety of all of our clients is always our first priority, and a client who is abusing drugs and alcohol presents a danger to himself and those around him. For those clients who were previously weekend drinkers, the extra leisure time in their lives invites imbibing more often. Some clients say they drink because they are in pain. When further questioned about taking the prescribed anti-inflammatory, they say they are not taking it because they are not supposed to take it with alcohol and they would rather drink. This type of convoluted thinking is difficult to plow through successfully. Psychological counseling may help if the client is ready to take this step.

Currently, our work hardening center is staffed by all women, and there have been male clients who have arrived and announced that they do not take orders from women. At this point, the challenge has been issued. We immediately attempt to defuse the situation by explaining that we do not give orders. Our goal is to assist the client to reach his own goals. Further explanation of the program to make the client more comfortable in this environment also is attempted. It is extremely difficult to remain calm and understanding when being attacked. However, sensitivity to the client's background can aid in better handling the client's issues. A private discussion regarding the client's concerns with reassurance that we are not there to emasculate him but rather to assist in any way we can will help to set the tone for the entire program. If antisocial behavior, which is unacceptable, persists, the client may not be appropriate for the program at this time.

Clients also enter the work hardening program with fear of the unknown, fear of increasing pain, fear of improving and returning to the job, and fear of rejection in the job market when they are ready to return. Fear of the unknown can be addressed by providing a thorough orientation of exactly what the work hardening program entails (see Chapter 4).

When fear of improving and returning to work are issues, it is beneficial to try to gain knowledge of the client's underlying fears. Before injury, this worker was presumably a reliable, competent employee who had value to his company. His work provided an acceptable means to support himself and his family. So why would he be afraid to return? The reasons include fear of harassment by co-workers and management, being placed in a job exceeding his limits, being fired, and working with pain or discomfort. A couple of injured workers recently were terrified to go back into the workplace, and they experienced sleeplessness, nightmares, and physical illness any time they went inside the plant. The psychologist diagnosed post-traumatic stress disorder, a problem we more frequently associate with war veterans. In severe cases such as these, a combination of counseling and physical rehabilitation is most successful.

The self-esteem associated with being a fruitful, contributing member of society takes a beating when injured workers are out of work for extended periods of time. Along with the plunging self-esteem is the weight gain that accompanies inactivity and/or increased eating because of boredom or nervousness. The weight gain contributes to the low self-esteem. It is not unusual for this to become a self-perpetuating cycle leading to feelings of hopelessness and failure. Early intervention with an active program such as work hardening often can prevent the client from experiencing these negative repercussions. Weight gained is more readily lost with increased activity.

The client with low self-esteem may manifest feelings of anger, resentment, and uncooperativeness or may fall into self-pity. "Poor me. No one is going to want to hire me anymore. Besides, if I can't perform my physically demanding job like I used to, what good am I?" The self-pitying client is one of the most challenging clients to work with for those therapists who do not tolerate "poor me" very well. If possible, have a colleague work with the clients you have difficulty with. If nobody from your organization has the skills to work with a particular difficulty, share the responsibilities and, in the mean-time, seek a professional who can assist your group to gain the necessary skills. The clients also attend stress management classes that may assist to defuse some of the problem areas, and the professional providing stress management classes may be able to help you as well.

The obvious extreme of the worker displaying self-pity is the person who is truly depressed. There are degrees of depression. There is the person who just feels down, and there is the client who speaks openly about committing suicide. Always take the depressed client seriously when he speaks of suicide. Call the treating physician immediately to obtain an appointment for the client. Frequently, a course of antidepressants is helpful until the client assumes a more normal daily routine. Chemical imbalances do occur with a sudden, severe decrease in activity level, especially with the heavy laborer or the athlete. If the depression is not addressed, there can be serious consequences. At MPTC, no one has committed suicide, but the following example illustrates the consequences of ignored depression.

Paul was a 55-year-old man who was in a serious accident that resulted in many broken bones and bruised internal organs. He had been out of work for one year when he was referred to us. He was motivated and cooperative. He had a limited grade-school education and had been working for the local street department at the time of his injury. His job demanded physical labor, and it was highly unlikely that he would be able to return to this job. Paul's ability to understand written instructions was poor. Simple exercises and directions had to be reinstructed daily. He could not interpret pictures. Even with a therapist working closely with him, he could not retain appropriate techniques from day to day. Despite his difficulties, he was a pleasure to work with because he was so motivated and tried so hard to improve.

After about three weeks in the program, Paul began to express feelings of frustration, openly sharing his financial and family difficulties. His savings were almost gone and his wife had just had an abdominal operation. Because of his lack of understanding of medical terminology, he was not really sure exactly how serious her condition was. However, he perceived the situation at home to be serious. He said that he would be of more worth to his family if he committed suicide and they collected his life insurance. He could see no other way out. I called his physician and requested that the client be seen that day. The physician agreed. The client returned to work hardening the next day and acted as though everything was the same. He still spoke openly of shooting himself. I brought him to a private area where we could talk and questioned him about his visit to the physician the day before. He stated that the doctor had just wanted to see how he was doing in the program. Questioning further, I learned that the client and physician never even discussed the client's feelings of despair. No exchange had occurred at all! I called the physician to request his assessment of the client's mental state. He said that he saw no signs of depression but admitted that he had made no attempt to bring up the subject. When pressed further, the physician said that there was something definitely going on in the household because he was treating the client's 23-year-old son for depression. The son was still living at home and, until recently, had never experienced any emotional difficulties. The physician had been treating the entire family for more than 25 years and did not remember any previous pattern of depression. I urgently requested another visit for my client as he was to be discharged from the work hardening program shortly.

The problem was not resolved prior to the client's discharge. On subsequent follow-up, I learned that the depression continued to be ignored and no treatment was provided to the client. He eventually was committed to the state mental institute because he was suicidal and out of control.

This situation could have been avoided had the client been treated immediately before it became an emergency situation. The daily support system and stress management sessions held during work hardening are sometimes insufficient for the very depressed client. Recommendations for individual counseling are not well-received by the Workers' Compensation carrier in most cases. Although sometimes not the ideal, a visit to the treating physician and administration of antidepressants can be treatment enough to assist the depressed client.

There are probably as many different rehabilitation scenarios played out across the country as there are injured workers. There is absolutely no way to prepare for all of them. Each new incident should be treated as a learning experience. Take your time in deciding how to handle each challenge. The first time a client yelled at me because he was angry that he had to be in work hardening, I was dumbstruck. It was obvious that I was the recipient of some displaced anger. Fortunately for me, we were alone in the center at the time. I left the room and told the client that we both needed some time to reflect. Fifteen minutes later, we sat down together and discussed what he was feeling. He did fine after that day. He graduated from the program two weeks later and successfully returned to his original job. I knew right away that I needed to contract a professional to assist these depressed and angry clients on their road to recovery.

For those who are new to working with this population, the following list of common quotes may help you to prepare for when the client says:

1. "I'm in such pain, I can't come in today."
2. "Assessment made me worse."
3. "Exercises are making me worse, so I'm seeing my doctor today. I'm not coming in!"
4. (If the client is working too fast)—"But this is how I always work." (Working too slow)—"I'm afraid to do too much. I don't work this hard at my job."
5. "My wife/husband says I shouldn't have to do this because it's making me worse!"
6. "I have to watch the kids today."
7. "My child has a ball game. I have to go."
8. "I have an appointment with my attorney, so I won't be in today."
9. "I have to get back to work or I'll lose my home."
10. "My daughter was beat up last night, and I'm upset."
11. "I don't want to quit drinking!" "I drink because of the pain."
12. "I'm bored with this program."
13. "I don't take orders from women!"
14. "What if I cannot go back to my job?" "What good am I?"
15. "No one is going to want to hire me."
16. "I'm going to shoot myself!"
17. "I'm not sleeping at night, so I can't come in consistently."
18. "I've gained 50 pounds."
19. "My car broke down. I don't have transportation. I won't be in until I do."
20. "I can't read well so how can I follow this program?"

Some of the things we hear are very appropriate reasons not to attend at least for that day. With those clients who do not have any direction or have difficulty establishing goals, the reasons for not committing to the work hardening program are lame excuses that we do not accept. Poor excuses for not attending are as much a reason for discharge as not showing up at the client's scheduled appointment time.

At MPTC we treat each case individually. There are some facilities where a certain number of cancellations means automatic discharge. Each organization must decide what its own policy will be. Whenever a client is discharged for noncompliance with the program, we always make it clear to the client that his insurance company is one of the parties that will receive a copy of the discharge notes which will state the reason for discharge as noncompliance. Although we are not trying to establish an adversarial role with the client, it is imperative that he understand his responsibility to make every attempt to improve and return to the workforce and the consequences if he chooses not to do so.

CHAPTER 4

Entering the
Work Hardening Program

Now that we know the appropriate candidates for admission into work hardening, we will trace the admission process. The client is referred to the center by someone familiar with the injured worker's case. The initial appointment is made through the referral source or directly with the client, and the intake record is filled out (Figure 4–1). If the client has not yet had an FCA, one is scheduled. When functional capabilities are ascertained, the work hardening process begins.

The client is scheduled for day one and is sent our Work Hardening Orientation booklet (Figure 4–2). This provides him with generic information about the program. The purpose of this booklet is to allay any anxieties and fear of the unknown. The client is encouraged to read the booklet and to make note of any questions or concerns that arise during its reading.

ORIENTATION

Upon arrival for his scheduled appointment, the client is greeted by the therapist who will be working with him on that day. He will receive one-to-one attention to acclimate him to his new surroundings. The therapist and client review the contents of the Work Hardening Orientation booklet together. The client again receives a brief explanation of the results of his FCA (a full explanation should have been provided prior to this day). Any questions the client has are addressed during the orientation process. The client is provided with a definition of work hardening. Be prepared to receive some resistance to discussion of return to work from some of your clients, especially from those clients who are somewhat focused on the continuing discomfort accompanying their injury. Successful completion of the work hardening program is not dependent on the client's immediate acceptance of the idea. Keeping his whole life in perspective, including his need to develop a comfort level with all aspects of his life again, will eventually lead to acceptance of his role in the workplace.

During orientation, the client learns about his rights and his responsibilities under the Workers' Compensa-

tion law of Maine. The treating therapist thus must have a working knowledge of the Workers' Compensation law. The laws are different in each state. You can obtain a copy of your law by calling or writing the Workers' Compensation office in your state. A list of the most current names and addresses of these offices is provided in the Appendix. Do not be overwhelmed by the size of the book when you receive it. Every aspect of the law is included. It is not necessary for you to gain a full understanding of everything stated within the law. The most important parts to learn are those involved in the rehabilitation section. Clients will enter your work-hardening program with little or no understanding of how the system works. With the knowledge the treating therapist can impart, clients frequently relax and begin to trust. Such tidbits as mileage reimbursement for medical appointments may allow the client with financial difficulty to attend work hardening with less stress. Anything we can do to decrease stress levels will assist the client to improve more quickly.

The orientation process also provides time to discuss available classes such as back school, healthy upper-body training, stress management classes, and general stretching techniques.

The clients are encouraged to begin setting goals that are both personal and job- or career-related. The shift back to self-reliance and control over one's own life begins with goal setting, otherwise known in some centers as "goaling." Goaling can be a very difficult process for injured workers who have been without control for months or longer. The therapist will need to demonstrate restraint if the client is having difficulty setting goals. The impulse is to make suggestions. Nevertheless, we must resist this because the client is certain to assume the goals suggested by the therapist, pretending they are his own. In reality, the client may not have any idea what he wants to gain from work hardening or where he wants to go from here. I heard a colleague speaking to a group of professionals recently regarding the "how to's" of setting up a work hardening center. I was most struck by the lecturer's apparent disregard for the client's need to have some control over his own future.

INTAKE RECORD

☐ FCA ☐ WH   Ref. Rec'd. _____/_____/_____

                                                          Referred By: _____

Client: _____ Phone #: _____

Address: _____ DOB: _____

_____

Diagnosis: _____

D.O.I.: _____/_____/_____   Medical Hx Req.: _____

Insurance Company: _____

Address: _____

_____

Adjuster: _____ Phone #: _____

Employer: _____

Address: _____

_____

Voc. Rehab. Counselor: _____

Name of Company: _____

Address: _____ Phone #: _____

_____

Insurance Approval: ☐ Yes   ☐ No

If No, Reason: _____

_____

Date of Approval: FCA _____/_____/_____   WH _____/_____/_____

Name and Title of Person Approving: _____

Client Preparation: 1) Clothing/Shoes ☐

                           2) Eye Glasses   ☐

Scheduled Appointment: _____/_____/_____

Figure 4–1. Sample Intake Record for Functional Capacity Assessments and Work Hardening Referrals

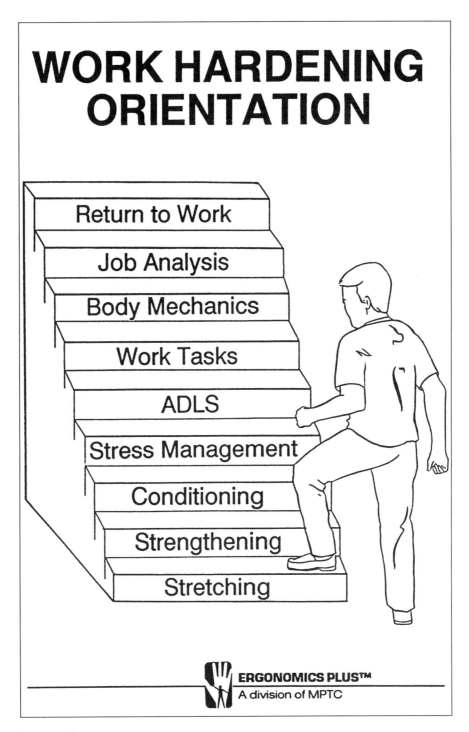

Figure 4–2.

The speaker constantly spoke of the therapist's goals for his clients. The injured worker measures his successes by the achievement of his goals, not the therapist's goals for him. When the client appears unable to establish goals and we know that this is an important part of the client's return to self-reliance, the treating therapist must seek

out methods of stimulating the goal-setting process. If a professional colleague is unavailable on site, then a contract person with experience in this area should be consulted. Five to 10 goals should be obtained during orientation because this provides much insight into the client's plans for the future. Realistically, we just obtain what we can and at least begin the process of thinking toward the future. Goals become real once they are written down.

A pain drawing (Figure 4–3) to provide the treating therapist with information regarding specificity of complaints and, therefore, the possibility of the presence of symptom magnification is completed during orientation. The pain drawing should reflect the area of injury and not cover the entire body! A client once arrived for an initial assessment with a completed pain drawing blown up to cover three sheets of paper taped together! She had not been asked to provide any of this information. Prior to assessment we always receive objective medical records. However, beyond that, we like to enter the assessment process unbiased. An injured worker who needs a pain drawing this large in order to have space to note all of the codes has certainly lost perspective of the original problem somewhere along the way. The benefit of knowing that this may be the case before starting work hardening is to direct the program right away to defocus on the client's complaints and refocus on his capabilities. In an indirect way, we already do that in work hardening just by its set-up, but with the pain-focused client, a more direct approach is absolutely imperative.

Although a job analysis is the most accurate method of obtaining a description of the injured worker's job tasks, performing a job analysis is not always possible prior to the initiation of work hardening. Consequently, we developed the job description questionnaire (Figures 4–4 through 4–6). The client answers all questions to the best of his ability. The answers are not always totally accurate but do provide a sense of the job and further insight into the client's relationship with his employer. Another avenue for obtaining this information is to request a job description from the company. If you are fortunate enough to receive this in a timely manner, take some time to scrutinize it. These are not totally accurate either. Job descriptions are written as vaguely and incompletely as possible to permit task flexibility within the company's workforce. Nevertheless, until a site visit is permitted to obtain a first-hand job analysis, the above methods are helpful.

Finally, a brief neuromusculoskeletal screening is performed (Figure 4–7). Although the work hardening program is functionally focused, specific musculoskeletal deficits do interfere with the client's progress. With the screening, we find these problems early on and build a work hardening schedule to address all issues at the same time. The screening also provides further insight into the client's agenda. For example, if during a gross testing of the quadriceps musculature we get a cogwheel release pattern without the presence of ap-propriate illness, there is reason to suspect psychological overlay. Complaints and testing that do not follow a dermatomal or myotomal pattern are other clues to the client's attitude.

General information dispensed during orientation to the client provides guidelines for a successful recovery. These guidelines are:

1. Expect a certain amount of soreness or increase in discomfort. If this does not happen, fine. But oftentimes, the increase in activity level does increase discomfort.
2. If you notice that a specific exercise or activity causes increased discomfort, report it. We will work with you to find a better way.
3. Do not change anything about your program before consulting with the therapist. If you increase on your own, you may exceed your recognized safe parameters.
4. Daily attendance is required. Successful progress in work hardening is dependent on consistency. It is best to treat your program as if it was your job. If you are ill and cannot attend, a telephone call is required.
5. Avoid caffeine. Caffeine and nicotine can increase your symptoms. We serve decaffeinated beverages at this facility.
6. If you are here through lunchtime, a refrigerator and microwave are available for your use in the lunchroom.
7. Use of assistive devices is allowed while participating in the work hardening program. The therapist will help you put them on and take them off if necessary.
8. There are hot packs, cold packs, and ice massage popsicles available. You must identify when and if you need them.
9. Stress management classes are held twice a week for 45 minutes each time. Attendance is required. In a group setting, this is your opportunity to problem solve with an objective facilitator regarding issues that are important to you.

The list of information you provide at your facility may be different. The object of having this information written down somewhere is that the client can refer back to it whenever he feels that it is necessary. Clients become overwhelmed with input during the orientation process and do not remember everything.

The orientation process establishes the tone for the entire work hardening experience. At the completion of orientation, the injured worker has a picture of what to expect from the facility and of what his responsibilities are toward his recovery. It is hoped that the client's anxiety level has improved with knowing what this unique program has to offer him. The individuality of each client's program provides the

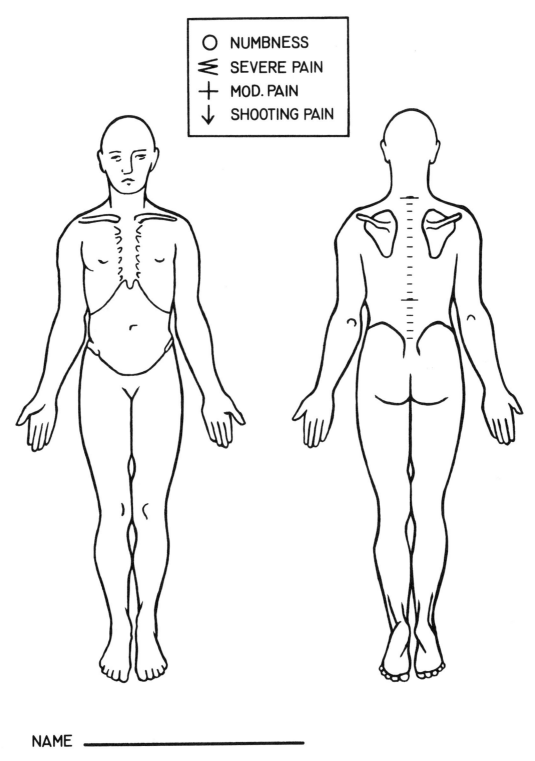

NAME ————————————————

Figure 4–3.

opportunity for the client to be an active participator right from the beginning. The client is introduced to the work hardening environment and equipment.

If he lifts buckets for a living, he will lift buckets during his program. He can identify with this and it feels "normal."

(*text continues on page 55*)

JOB DESCRIPTION QUESTIONNAIRE

Name: _____ Date: _____

What is your specific job title?_____

How many hours do you work per day?_____ week _____ overtime _____?

Do you have breaks?   ☐ Yes   ☐ No

   give specifics _____

Please try to answer all questions which pertain to your past job, or job you would like to go to after Work Hardening.

1. Do you incorporate any of these activities during your work day?

	YES	NO	HOW LONG?
a. drive	☐	☐	_____
b. walk	☐	☐	_____
c. stair climb	☐	☐	_____
d. sit	☐	☐	_____
e. twist	☐	☐	_____
f. stand	☐	☐	_____
g. bend over	☐	☐	_____
h. squat	☐	☐	_____
i. kneel	☐	☐	_____
j. reach	☐	☐	_____

2. Do you incorporate any pushing/pulling?   ☐ Yes   ☐ No

   If yes, please answer the following:

   a. What do you push/pull_____

   _____

   b. How far?_____

   c. How much weight is involved?_____

   d. What type of surface to you push/pull across?_____

   _____

   e. Does the unit have wheels?   ☐ Yes   ☐ No

   f. Which picture best describes you when you push?

   g. Comments: _____

   _____

Figure 4–4.   Blank Job Description Questionnaire for Readers Use in their Facility

JOB DESCRIPTION QUESTIONNAIRE

3. Do you incorporate any lifting?   ☐ Yes   ☐ No

   If yes, please answer the following:

   a. What do you lift? _____

   _____

   b. How many pounds is it? (please explain if the weight varies) _____

   _____

   c. What distance is your lift? (example: ground level to shoulder level)_____

   _____

   d. Comments: _____

4. Does your job require any carrying?   ☐ Yes   ☐ No

   If yes, please answer the following:

   a. What type of object(s) do you carry? _____

   _____

   b. How much weight do you carry and how far? _____

   _____

   c. What do you carry with? (example: hand, mechanical equipment, basket)_____

   d. Does the weight vary? _____

5. Do you use any special equipment (jackhammer, computers, forklift, saws, machinery)?

   Please explain: _____

   _____

6. Are you right or left handed?_____

7. Task Description - briefly explain:

   a. repetitive motions performed_____

   _____

   b. describe materials you handle_____

   _____

   c. production oriented (piece or incentive work)_____

   _____

   d. quota standards_____

   _____

8. Demonstration***

Figure 4–4.   (continued)

JOB DESCRIPTION QUESTIONNAIRE

Name: ___Ben D. Nees_____   Date:___4-26_____

What is your specific job title?___warehouse worker_____

How many hours do you work per day?___8___ week ___40___ overtime _____?

Do you have breaks? ☑Yes ☐No

give specifics ___2 - 15 min. and 1/2 hour lunch_____

Please try to answer all questions which pertain to your past job, or job you would like to go to after Work Hardening.

1. Do you incorporate any of these activities during your work day?

	YES	NO	HOW LONG?
a. drive	☑	☐	
b. walk	☑	☐	
c. stair climb	☑	☐	
d. sit	☑	☐	
e. twist	☑	☐	
f. stand	☑	☐	
g. bend over	☑	☐	
h. squat	☑	☐	
i. kneel	☑	☐	
j. reach	☑	☐	shelves are 2 ft. deep

2. Do you incorporate any pushing/pulling? ☑Yes ☐No

If yes, please answer the following:

a. What do you push/pull___hand trucks loaded with food_____

b. How far?___up to 30 feet_____

c. How much weight is involved?___200 lbs._____

d. What type of surface to you push/pull across?___cement floor_____

e. Does the unit have wheels? ☑Yes ☐No

f. Which picture best describes you when you push?

g. Comments: _____

Figure 4–5. Sample Completed Job Description Questionnaire for Low Back Injured Patient

JOB DESCRIPTION QUESTIONNAIRE

3. Do you incorporate any lifting? ☑Yes ☐No

   If yes, please answer the following:

   a. What do you lift? __boxed food__

   b. How many pounds is it? (please explain if the weight varies) __50 - 75 lbs.__

   c. What distance is your lift? (example: ground level to shoulder level)__from floor to chest level off from__ __floor to overhead (10' ceilings)__

   d. Comments:_____

4. Does your job require any carrying? ☑Yes ☐No

   If yes, please answer the following:

   a. What type of object(s) do you carry? __boxed food and groceries__

   b. How much weight do you carry and how far? __50 - 75 lbs. up to 30 feet__

   c. What do you carry with? (example: hand, mechanical equipment, basket)__forklift, hand truck, and hand__

   d. Does the weight vary? __yes__

5. Do you use any special equipment (jackhammer, computers, forklift, saws, machinery)?

   Please explain: __forklift, hand truck, and ladders__

6. Are you right or left handed?__right__

7. Task Description - briefly explain:

   a. repetitive motions performed__carrying, bending throughout the day__

   b. describe materials you handle__boxes of dry goods or produce (occasionally 40°-50° temperatures__

   c. production oriented (piece or incentive work)__below__

   d. quota standards__below__

Addendum from the Client:
The company has instituted a new system in which each employee is expected to produce a certain amount of work in a given time period. Mr. Nees finds it very difficult to keep up with the younger people and finds the time systems quite unfair. Even though there are aisles that contain lighter groceries, Mr. Nees says it is not possible to take purchase orders that involve work in the lighter aisles. This is "unfair to other employees," and they would "frown on it." In order to meet the "time limits," he feels it is not practical to use step ladders. The company has provided wheeled stools that secure themselves with weight bearing. However, the client feels these are dangerous when lifting overhead if standing on the edge of the stool and therefore refuses to use them. Mr. Nees also feels that it would take "too much time" to use proper body mechanics while loading pallets.

Figure 4–5. (continued)

JOB DESCRIPTION QUESTIONNAIRE

Name: _____Carrie Proppa_____ Date:___7-28_____

What is your specific job title?_____quality operator "Inspector"_____

How many hours do you work per day?____8_____ week ___40____ overtime _____?

Do you have breaks?   ☑Yes   ☐No
     give specifics ____2 - 15 min. and 1/2 hour lunch_____

Please try to answer all questions which pertain to your past job, or job you would like to go to after Work Hardening.

1. Do you incorporate any of these activities during your work day?

	YES	NO	HOW LONG?
a. drive	☑	☐	1/2 hour to/from work
b. walk	☑	☐	during breaks
c. stair climb	☐	☑	
d. sit	☑	☐	all day
e. twist	☐	☑	
f. stand	☐	☑	as needed
g. bend over	☐	☑	
h. squat	☐	☑	
i. kneel	☐	☑	
j. reach	☑	☐	shelves are 2 ft. deep

2. Do you incorporate any pushing/pulling?   ☐ Yes   ☑No

    If yes, please answer the following:

    a. What do you push/pull____hand trucks loaded with food_____

    b. How far?____up to 30 feet_____

    c. How much weight is involved?____200 lbs._____

    d. What type of surface to you push/pull across?___cement floor_____

    e. Does the unit have wheels?   ☑Yes   ☐No

    f. Which picture best describes you when you push?

    g. Comments: _____

Figure 4–6.   Sample Completed Job Description Questionnaire for Upper Extremity Injured Client

JOB DESCRIPTION QUESTIONNAIRE

3. Do you incorporate any lifting? ☑ Yes   ☐ No

   If yes, please answer the following:

   a. What do you lift? __boxes of circuits__

   b. How many pounds is it? (please explain if the weight varies) __20-30 lbs.__

   c. What distance is your lift? (example: ground level to shoulder level)__from floor to the level I work at__

   d. Comments:_____

4. Does your job require any carrying?   ☑ Yes   ☐ No

   If yes, please answer the following:

   a. What type of object(s) do you carry? __boxes of circuits__

   b. How much weight do you carry and how far? __20-30 lbs. across room about 20 feet__

   c. What do you carry with? (example: hand, mechanical equipment, basket)__hand__

   d. Does the weight vary? __yes__

5. Do you use any special equipment (jackhammer, computers, forklift, saws, machinery)?

   Please explain: __special chairs are provided__

6. Are you right or left handed?__right__

7. Task Description - briefly explain:

   a. repetitive motions performed__constant two-handed twisting up and down a circuit board__

   b. describe materials you handle__circuit switches, circuit boxes__

   c. production oriented (piece or incentive work)__none__

   d. quota standards_____

8. Demonstration***

Figure 4–6. (continued)

PHYSICAL THERAPY MUSCLE IMBALANCE SUMMARY

Patient Name: _____

Diagnosis/Assessment: _____

Date: _____/_____/_____

Subjective: _____

_____

Objective: _____

_____

Postural/Imbalance Deficits

Head	_____ Forward				
Shoulders	_____ Forward	_____ Flat			
Thoracic	_____ Kyphosis	_____ Flat			
Lumbar	_____ Flat	_____ Lordosis			
Pelvic Tilt	_____ Anterior	_____ Posterior			
Knees	_____ Valgus	_____ Varus	_____ Hyperextended		
Ankles	_____ Supinated	_____ Pronated			
Toes	_____ Hallux Valgus	_____ MP Hyperextended	_____ Hammer		

T = Tight Muscles   W = Weak Muscles

_____	Iliopsoas	_____	Pectoralis Minor
_____	Quadriceps	_____	Shoulder Internal Rotator
_____		_____	External Abdominal Oblique
_____	TFL	_____	Gastrocsoleus
_____		_____	Hip Extensor
_____	Hamstrings	_____	Toe Extensor
_____		_____	Anterior Tibialis

ROM/Strength Extremities

UE		Right	Left	ROM/Cervical/Thoracic/Lumbar/Spine
SHOULDER	Flexion	_____	_____	_____
	Abduction	_____	_____	_____
	Internal Rotation	_____	_____	_____
	External Rotation	_____	_____	_____
	Adduction	_____	_____	_____
ELBOW	Flexion	_____	_____	_____
	Extension	_____	_____	_____
WRIST	Flexion	_____	_____	_____
	Extension	_____	_____	_____
	Supination	_____	_____	_____
	Pronation	_____	_____	_____
	Grip Strength	_____	_____	_____

Therapist_____

Figure 4–7. Sample Muscle Screening Tool for Work Hardening Entry

To avoid any misconceptions the client's spouse may have about the program, to provide support to the client, or just to develop a general comfort level with the entire family, the client's spouse is invited to visit the facility to observe the client in his program. During this scheduled visit, the therapist answers any questions the spouse may have and supplies a full explanation of the concept of work hardening. Of course, this is not mandatory, but it does reflect the philosophy of the facility to support the client in any way possible to ensure his successful completion of the program. There is no doubt that a work injury affects the entire family, not just the client.

WRITING THE WORK HARDENING PROGRAM

Prior to the orientation process, the therapist has reviewed all of the information gathered during prior treatments and during the FCA. The baseline information that is reviewed first is FCA results. We look at the workday tolerance—how many hours per day and duration of activities. What are position tolerances? For example, can he bend, stoop, crouch, crawl, and kneel? If so, how often and how long? What kind of resistance can he safely tolerate? Can he lift, carry, push, and pull? If so, how much, how often, for how long, from which levels? What were the recommendations of the assessment specialist for this client? Were there any ancillary observations stated in the recommendations that would provide insight into this client's needs?

It is critical to the safety of the client to note any limitations present when establishing a work hardening schedule and not to exceed those limits when beginning the program. The goal of the program is to begin at a safe level, and then progress beyond that level as the client makes gains. The "occasional," "frequent," and "continuous" limitations are probably the most difficult parameters to adhere to at first. Accepted definitions of these terms are:

Occasional— 1 to 33% of the workday;
Up to 20 nonconsecutive minutes per hour;
Performed less than once every three minutes

Frequent— 34 to 66% of the workday;
Up to 40 nonconsecutive minutes per hour;
One or more times every three minutes up to one hour

Continuous—67 to 100% of the workday;
Continuously for eight hours;
One or more times per three minutes for more than one hour

At the completion of the functional assessment, these limits (or, looking on the more positive side, these remaining capabilities) should be delineated clearly for the client's safety. We are indeed fortunate that occupational rehabilitation has come this far to provide us with this important information. Nevertheless, all of this information can appear overwhelming to the new work hardening provider. Proper training in establishing safe work hardening programs based on this information is recommended strongly. This type of therapy approach rarely is discussed as part of the basic education that therapists receive. However, many educators plan to change that. Until then or for further insight, taking a good "how to" course is recommended.

After studying the FCA results, a review of the medical records is helpful. This information reiterates the course of treatment and triggers any missed points that the therapist may feel compelled to follow-up. Any referral for a work hardening program should be scrutinized for appropriateness. A review of care sometimes reveals a need to instigate alternative treatment or further investigate the cause of continued signs and symptoms.

A client profile is helpful when available. Unfortunately, this type of information frequently does not surface until well after the treatment has begun. Such information includes marital status, presence and number of children at home, comfort of home and living arrangements, and presence of social difficulties either directly involving the client or within his family. Circumstances such as a dependent parent living within the home or an independent parent who lives alone but has Alzheimer's disease create stressors that may inhibit the ability of the client to improve. Knowing some of these circumstances prior to the inception of the program, the therapist may be able to schedule the client to enable him to meet his personal obligations more easily. This can be a real consideration especially when the injured worker had worked the evening or night shift in order to ease the burden of care at home. Most work hardening centers do not function around the clock and cannot totally simulate the client's work habits. We always tell the clients that they should treat their work hardening treatment as though it is the job that Workers' Compensation is paying them to do. But this can be difficult for clients with special needs.

Although the information exchanged during stress management sessions is confidential, the stress management provider may be able to provide generic client profile information for the treating therapist to aid the client's recovery. Usually if the treating therapist has not been informed of problems at home, the information will surface during stress management sessions. Another avenue is to have the stress management therapist encourage the client to share the information with his work hardening therapist. There always should be a private space available for the client to have some personal time with the therapist when needed.

With the information from all of these sources, the work hardening therapist can write an initial work hardening program. Most of our clients begin their programs at only two hours per day. Unfortunately, this does not leave much time for work simulation at the onset of the program. However, during the stretching, strengthening, body mechanics, and education classes, the therapist observes the client's abilities and willingness to participate actively in his own care. This brief interval of the treatment process permits the treating therapist to gather more job information that can be integrated as the client's hours increase in the program. As the client's job is broken down methodically into its component parts, the client increases the number of hours per day he is spending at the work hardening center. Because the work hardening approach is to train the injured worker to return to his job using the same or similar tasks as are performed at the worksite, introduction to job tasks should be initiated by the second week in the program. By this time, it is rare to have a client who is spending less than four hours per day with you.

Punching a Clock

All work hardening programs should include those responsibilities inherent in the world of gainful employment as well as those components necessary to facilitate the client's physical recovery. All clients begin by punching a time clock. This assures timeliness and is one method of keeping accurate records of such. Some clients think nothing of coming in five or ten minutes late. Once they have begun to punch a clock and realize that this is more like working than rehabilitation, they become more serious with their timeliness. This is a critical component to the client's successful return to the workforce.

Clipboard Program

To facilitate independence, the client's program is placed on a clipboard hanging within the center. The client reports to work hardening by punching the clock and retrieving his clipboard from the wall. He reviews the day's program and discusses any changes or any questions he has with the therapist. At our facility, we indicate program changes by color blocking that activity for that day because otherwise the complacent client who has become accustomed to his program does not pick up the changes when they are assigned. This does not accomplish what was intended in the time frame in

which it was intended. You can use whatever works for your clientele.

Stretching

Our work hardening clients stretch at the beginning of their workday. We are trying to facilitate a better sense of body awareness. Most clients have been in abnormal postures and have been using compensatory muscle groups and protecting the injured area for so long that they have forgotten what the body felt like prior to injury. The slow, deliberate stretching movements not only increase the client's flexibility so they can move better but also provide body awareness input. The stretching program is kept to a reasonable length of time as this is a task that we are trying to make habitual. Clients receive a copy of their stretching program for home use as soon as we are confident that they have a full understanding of the proper techniques. "Mini" stretch breaks are taught early in the program as an injury-control mechanism. These minibreaks are changes in posture to return the muscle groups that are used most frequently back to their normal length. We teach our clients that fatigue of musculature is a warning that a 10-second stretch is indicated.

Cardiovascular Activities

Cardiovascular activities are included in everyone's program regardless of the area of injury. Any injury results in a decreased activity level that leads to decreased cardiovascular endurance. Everyone who works has developed a certain level of endurance to maintain the job position. During work hardening, we do not need to condition the injured worker to the level of an elite athlete, but the client must regain the endurance to comfortably return to the job. I "work out" at the local health club four days per week. When I go away on a business trip for several days, my cardiovascular endurance drops if I cannot find a place to work out. When I return, I must start back at a lower level than when I left and work back up. The injured worker functions much the same. Another issue to consider is the circulatory compromise in areas of injury where spasm and immobility have prevailed. Challenging the cardiovascular system assists to increase general endurance as well as to bring circulation to previously compromised areas.

Body Mechanics

Body mechanics and postural re-education are integral components of the work hardening program. Although classes are an excellent method of introducing the information all at once, the ongoing reinforcement of learned techniques assures the client's safety on the job by making the correct movements habitual. The only way for this to occur is to reinforce the techniques every day. Once job tasks have been identified, the client's program can be written to integrate the necessary movements to practice without being contrived. This more natural environment makes it easier for the client to relate. Along with the work movements, the client also should have the opportunity to perform movements involved in his daily tasks. For example, one of the biggest motivators for improvement with a back-injured client may be the desire to pick up his two-year-old child. To accomplish this goal, while gaining the ability to return to work, creates a balance for the client between home and work. The client who is nervous about returning to work may respond better initially performing tasks more related to activities of daily living (ADLs). Just be cautious that this does not happen for longer than a week or so. By then, specific work-related tasks should begin.

Normal Workday

Once the client begins to increase the time spent at the work hardening center, it becomes necessary to integrate normal workday breaks into his routine. Generally, breaks are 15 minutes for the four-hour client; 15 minutes in the morning and 30 minutes for lunch for the six-hour client; and the eight-hour client has 15 minutes in the morning and afternoon and 30 minutes for lunch. The time clock can be used in your center for all breaks if you think it is what you need to facilitate timeliness. We usually have the clients punch in and out at lunchtime.

Circuits

The client's "productivity circuits" are the structured introductions to specific work tasks, especially as they relate to productivity (Figures 4–8 through 4–11). Prior to composing appropriate circuits for each client, a full breakdown of the client's job into its component tasks must be completed, using a "job analysis" form (Figures 4–12 through 4–17). Summaries of the client's job analysis are then sent to his physician (Figures 4–18 and 4–19).

A task may be something as simple as "lift the box weighing two pounds from the floor." The next step may be to carry it 10 feet. Another task would be to place the box on the conveyer belt. This is a very simplistic task breakdown, but if the client cannot safely perform any one of these duties, the job must be broken into

small enough components to allow him to begin job-task simulation. The job-task simulation performed during circuit training is one of the most important components of a true work hardening program. Job-task simulation provides the opportunity to identify any potential problem tasks and to correct the problem in a supervised environment before returning to the job. It promotes the client's confidence in his ability to be productive at the worksite while, at the same time, equipping him with the necessary pain-control techniques to allow him to remain a functioning member of society. Our clients learn to work through the discomforts, learning which techniques work for them. We rarely allow the injured worker to omit a task that previously has been identified as safe. Complaints of discomfort are not acceptable grounds for avoiding a responsibility. Together with the client, the treating therapist works to identify an alternate method to allow completion of the task.

Social Dynamics

During the development of our work hardening program, the initiation of a weekly dynamic activity hour, or "dynohour," did not occur until several months into the program. Initially, the proper work environment in the work hardening center to stimulate development or redevelopment of necessary life skills appeared to be proceeding well in all areas except one. That one missing component was social skills. As you watch the dynamics of the clients in your center, you will notice that there are some groups who just naturally blend and cultivate relationships suitable to the work environment. But, because many times your clients are functioning on such different levels, this natural phenomenon may not occur. Therefore, the work hardening program must be set up to stimulate the social skills lost through months of isolation, fear, pain, and a myriad of other feelings. The work-injured client experiences a sudden loss of contact with all that is normal to him. The work hardening program is the path to return to more normal function. Thus, the dynohour was born. During this hour-long session, clients choose the activity as a group from a list of options based on the needs of the client population. Activities can be as benign as making a fruit salad to be shared at break time or as competitive as a game. Some examples of group dynamic hours are given in detail in Chapter One.

Teams can be formed or individuals can compete. If a competitive choice is made, care must be given to ensure that nobody leaves feeling like a loser. Despite the fact that it is only a game, injured workers who already feel discouraged take things very personally. If

(text continues on page 70)

Circuit

Occupation: Assembly Line Worker

Date	1-4	1-5	1-6	1-7	1-8	1-11	1-12	1-13	1-14
Hours	4 hrs.	4 hrs.	4 hrs.	4 hrs.	4 hrs.	6 hrs.	6 hrs.	6 hrs.	6 hrs.
Sorting (stand)	circular tiles	square tiles	red tiles	white tiles	circular tiles	square tiles	red tiles	white tiles	circular tiles
Desk Chair Lift	pivot 7#	pivot 7#	pivot 10#	pivot 10#	pivot 10#	pivot 13# •	pivot 13#	pivot 15#	pivot 15#
Minnesota	1/2 tray	1 tray	1 tray	1 1/2 trays	1 1/2 trays	2 trays	2 trays	2 1/2 trays •	2 1/2 trays
Push/Pull Cart	25 ft. 15#	25 ft. 20# •	25 ft. 20#	30 ft. 20# •	30 ft. 23# •	30 ft. 23#	35 ft. 25# •	35 ft. 25#	40 ft. 25# •
Flip Cards						1/2 deck	1/2 deck	1 deck •	1 deck
West II						level 3-5-8 10#	level 2-5-9 10# •	level 3-5-8 15# •	level 2-5-9 15# •
Deal Cards						1/2 deck	1/2 deck	1 deck•	1 deck
Bird Cage						level 2-4-6	level 3-7-9 •	level 2-4-6 •	level 3-7-9 •

Name_____Lucy Link_____

Figure 4–8. Sample Work Activity for Assembly Line Worker

Circuit

Occupation: Plumber

Date	6-6	6-7	6-6	6-9	6-10	6-13	6-14	6-15	6-16
Hours	4 hrs.	4 hrs.	4 hrs.	4 hrs.	4 hrs.	6 hrs.	6 hrs.	6 hrs.	6 hrs.
Push/Pull Cart	sled empty	sled +10# •	sled +10#	sled +12# •	sled +12#	sled +14# •	sled +14#	sled +17# •	sled +17#
Bucket Carry	15#	15#	17# •	17#	17#	19# •	19#	22# •	22#
West IV	level 2&6 tighten 1 screw	level 2&6 1 screw	level 2&6 1 screw	level 2&6 2 screws•	level 2&6 2 screws	level 2&6 2 screws	level 2&9 2 screws•	level 2&9 2 screws	level 2&6 2 screws
Brief Tool Use (BTU)	3 screws	3 screws	4 screws•	4 screws	4 screws	5 screws•	5 screws	5 screws	5 screws
Pipe Tree	3 joints	4 joints•	4 joints	5 joints•	5 joints	5 joints	6 joints•	6 joints	6 joints

Name_____ Paul Plumber _____

Figure 4-9. Sample Work Activity for Plumber

Circuit

Occupation: Florist

Date	5-2	5-3	5-4	5-5	5-6	5-9	5-10	5-11	5-12
Hours	4 hrs.	4 hrs.	4 hrs.	4 hrs.	4 hrs.	6 hrs.	6 hrs.	6 hrs.	6 hrs.
Tie Bows	2 bows	3 bows •	3 bows	4 bows •	4 bows	4 bows	4 bows	5 bows •	5 bows
Cut Flowers	5 stems	7 stems •	7 stems	7 stems	9 stems •	9 stems	9 stems	12 stems •	12 stems
Arrange Flowers	1 small arrange	1 small arrange	2 small arrange•	2 small arrange•	3 small arrange•	3 small arrange	3 small arrange	3 small arrange	3 small arrange
Adding Machine	add 1 column	add 1 column	add 2 columns•	add 2 columns	add 3 columns•	add 3 columns	add 3 columns	add 3 columns	add 3 columns
Top Soil						fill 1 pot	fill 2 pots •	fill 2 pots	fill 2 pots
Plant						1 pot	2 pots •	2 pots	2 pots
Mist & Water						1 pot	2 pots •	2 pots	2 pots
Floor - Knuckle Lift						15#	15#	18# •	18#

Name_____ Rose Flowers _____

Figure 4–10. Sample Work Activity for Florist

Circuit

Occupation: Drywaller

Date	3-7	3-8	3-9	3-10	3-11	3-14	3-15	3-16	3-17
Hours	4 hrs.	4 hrs.	4 hrs.	4 hrs.	4 hrs.	6 hrs.	6 hrs.	6 hrs.	6 hrs.
Push/Pull Sled (40#)	sled empty	sled +15# •	sled +15#	sled +25# •	sled +25#	sled +25#	sled +25#	sled +25#	sled +28# •
Wall Building	4 blocks	5 blocks •	5 blocks	7 blocks •	7 blocks	7 blocks	7 blocks	7 blocks	7 blocks
Walk n' Carry	10# B 25 ft.	10# B 25 ft.	10# B 35 ft. •	10# B 35 ft.	10# B 50 ft. •	10# B 50 ft.	10# B 50 ft.	10# B 55 ft. •	10# B 60 ft. •
Ceiling Sweep						30 ft.	35 ft. •	40 ft. •	45 ft. •
Carry						1/2 sheet drywall	1/2 sheet drywall	1 sheet drywall	1 sheet drywall
Floor Sweep						30 ft.	35 ft. •	40 ft. •	45 ft. •
Bucket Carry						15#	15#	17# •	17#

Name _____ Clay Carrier _____

Figure 4–11. Sample Work Activity for Drywaller

Name: _____   Date:_____

Diagnosis: _____   Employer:_____

Job Title: _____   Work Hours: _____ Breaks: _____

Job Description: _____

_____

_____

Equipment Used: _____

Amount Spent: Sitting _____%   Standing _____%   Walking _____%

Employee Required to:	Yes	No	Time	Distance	Weight
A. Bend	☐	☐	_____	_____	_____
B. Squat	☐	☐	_____	_____	_____
C. Crawl	☐	☐	_____	_____	_____
D. Climb Stairs	☐	☐	_____	_____	_____
E. Kneel	☐	☐	_____	_____	_____
F. Crouch	☐	☐	_____	_____	_____

Employee Required to:	Yes	No	Time	Distance	Weight
Lift Above Shoulder	☐	☐	_____	_____	_____
Lift Desk/Chair	☐	☐	_____	_____	_____
Lift Chair/Floor	☐	☐	_____	_____	_____
Carry	☐	☐	_____	_____	_____
Repetitive Foot Movement	☐	☐	_____	_____	_____
Repetitive Hand Movement	☐	☐	_____	_____	_____
Repetitive Neck Movement	☐	☐	_____	_____	_____
Can Job Be Modified	☐	☐	_____		

Figure 4–12.   Sample Job Analysis Data Sheet for Use in Reader's Facility

Name: _____David Woods_____   Date: ____June 15, 1900____

Diagnosis: ____low back pain____   Employer: ____Maine Paper Co.____

Job Title: ____chip dumping operator____   Work Hours: __40/wk__ Breaks: ____1/2____

Job Description: ____stands at control panel pushing buttons which activates chip-dump____

_____

_____

Equipment Used: ____control panel____

Amount Spent: Sitting ____25____%   Standing ____50____%   Walking ____25____%

Employee Required to:	Yes	No	Time	Distance	Weight
A. Bend	☐	☑			
B. Squat	☐	☑			
C. Crawl	☐	☑			
D. Climb Stairs	☑	☐	4x	11 steps	
E. Kneel	☐	☑			
F. Crouch	☐	☑			

Employee Required to:	Yes	No	Time	Distance	Weight
Lift Above Shoulder	☐	☑			
Lift Desk/Chair	☐	☑			
Lift Chair/Floor	☐	☑			
Carry	☐	☑			
Repetitive Foot Movement	☐	☑			
Repetitive Hand Movement	☑	☐			
Repetitive Neck Movement	☑	☐			
Can Job Be Modified	☑	☐	sit/stand/walk as needed		

Figure 4–13. Sample Completed Job Analysis Data Sheet for Client with Low Back Pain

Name: _____   Date:_____

Diagnosis: _____   Employer:_____

Job Title: _____,   Work Hours: _____ Breaks: _____

Job Description: _____

_____

_____

Equipment Used: _____

Amount Spent: Sitting _____%   Standing _____%   Walking _____%

WORK STATION MEASUREMENTS:

Seat

A = Seat Tilt

D = Seat Depth

H = Seat Height

Back Rest Height

Back Rest Tilt

W = Seat Width

Easily Adjustable?

Desk

H = Height

D = Depth

W = Width

HT = Height to Terminal (eye level)

B = Keyboard Position

Others   90/90?

Arms on Chair?

Feet Firmly on floor?

Figure 4–14.   Sample Blank Job Analysis Data Sheet #2 for Use in Reader's Facility

Name: _____ Mary Jones _____   Date: ____ March 6, 1988 _____

Diagnosis: _____ right wrist tendinitis _____   Employer: ___ Strait N. Teeth, DDS _____

Job Title: _____ orthodontic technician _____   Work Hours: _50/wk_ Breaks: _1 hr. lunch____
                                                                                    2- 1/2 hr. breaks

Job Description: ___ uses pliers to bend wires, paints on acrylic, trims acrylic with a grinder _____

_____

_____

Equipment Used: ___ grinder, pliers, paintbrush, knife, spatula _____

Amount Spent: Sitting __80___%   Standing __10___%   Walking __10___%

WORK STATION MEASUREMENTS:

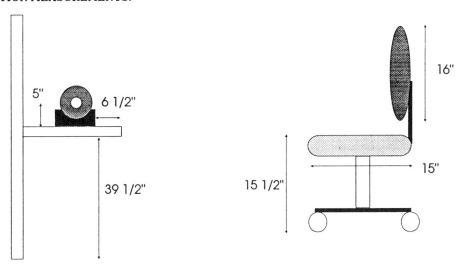

Seat			Desk		
A = Seat Tilt	none		H = Height	39 1/2"	
D = Seat Depth	15"		D = Depth	36"	
H = Seat Height	15 1/2"		W = Width	70"	
Back Rest Height			HT = Height to Terminal (eye level)		
Back Rest Tilt			B = Keyboard Position	(grinder)	
W = Seat Width			Others	90/90?	no
Easily Adjustable?	yes		Arms on Chair?	no	
			Feet Firmly on floor?		

Figure 4–15.   Sample Blank Job Analysis Data Sheet #2 for Patient with Wrist Tendinitis

Name: _____   Date: _____

Diagnosis: _____   Employer: _____

Job Title: _____   Work Hours: _____ Breaks: _____

Job Description: _____

_____

_____

Equipment Used: _____

Amount Spent: Sitting _____%   Standing _____%   Walking _____%

Lifting Measurements

(required to establish action limit and maximum permissible limit)

H – Horizontal location from midpoint between ankles to the center of the load at origin of lift (inches).

V – Vertical location of the hands at the beginning of the lift (floor to hands in inches).

D – Vertical distance from origin to destination of load (inches).

F – Average frequency of lift (lifts/minute).

$$AL \text{ (lbs.)} = 90(6/h)\,(1\text{-}.01/V\text{-}301)\,(.7 + 3/D)\,(1 - F/F_{max})$$

$$MPL = 3\,(AL)$$

Figure 4–16.   Sample Job Analysis Data Sheet for Use in Reader's Facility

Name: _____ A. King Back _____   Date: _____ January 2, 1991 _____

Diagnosis: _____ L4-5 Discectomy _____   Employer: _____

Job Title: _____ Material Handler _____   Work Hours: _40/wk_ Breaks: _____ 2-20 _____

Job Description: _____ lifts boxes of boxes to conveyor weight - 10# - 25# frequently _____

_____

_____

Equipment Used: _____ conveyor belt _____

Amount Spent: Sitting ____0____ %   Standing ____75____ %   Walking ____25____ %

Lifting Measurements

(required to establish action limit and maximum permissible limit)

H — Horizontal location from midpoint between ankles to the center of the load at origin of lift (inches).

V — Vertical location of the hands at the beginning of the lift (floor to hands in inches).

D — Vertical distance from origin to destination of load (inches).

F — Average frequency of lift (lifts/minute).

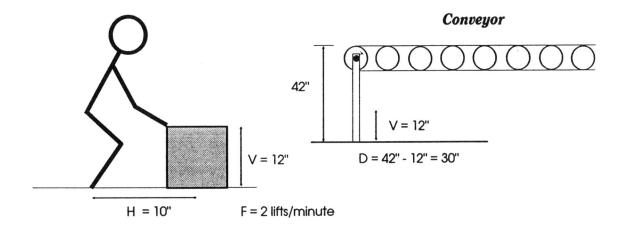

$$\text{AL (lbs.)} = 90(6/h)\,(1\text{-}.01/V\text{-}301)\,(.7 + 3/D)\,(1 - F/F_{max})$$

$$\text{MPL} = 3\,(\text{AL})$$

Figure 4–17. Sample Completed Job Analysis Data Sheet for Patient who is Post-Op L4-L5 discectomy with Job Title—Material Handler

June 15, 1988

Dr. KY Smith
ABC Lane
DEFGHI, JK 00000

RE: Job Analysis

Dear Dr. Smith:

I performed a Job Analysis on June 15, 1988, at _____. I observed the chip dumping operator position, which he/she will be returning to on June 24, 1988.

Based upon the Job Analysis, and his/her Assessment, I feel this job would be appropriate for him/her.

1. **Work Surface Height**
   Operator Position—30″ to 36″ from the floor.
   Assessment—Most comfortable work surface height reported to be between 36″ to 50″ from the floor.
   Recommendations—None

2. **Weight Required to Carry/Lift**
   Operator Position—None
   Present Lift Limit—35# occasionally
   Recommendations—Ask for assistance, if necessary, to lift any weights.

3. **Standing**
   Operating Position—Approximately 5 to 6 hours in an 8 hour workday.
   Assessment—3 to 4 hours in an 8 hour workday. 40 minute maximum durations.
   Recommendations—His/Her tolerance has increased for standing while participating in the Work Hardening Program. I do not anticipate he/she will have any difficulty with the standing required. If he does, there is a chair available for him to sit and also there is room for him to walk and do stretching.

4. **Chair**
   Operator Chair—The height of the chair is presently 25″ from the floor. The chair is not easily adjustable with poor lumbar support.
   Recommendations—Obtain a new chair which fits the following ergonomic guidelines.
   a. 4–5 prong base with swivel casters
   b. 10–11½″ back rest adjustable 2″
   c. Seat height 16″ to 22″ adjustable
   d. Front edge of seat with material that breathes
   e. Lumbar region that tilts at less than 80–120 degrees to give low back support.
   f. A foot rest on the bottom of the chair.

   To avoid low back strain from sitting consider:

   a. Sit in chair with hips and knees kept at right angles, feet flat on the floor.
   b. Utilize the entire sit with low back resting firmly on the low back rest.
   c. Use the foot rest to change positions and to eliminate stress on the low back.
   d. Change positions frequently by shifting weight or adjusting the chair.
   e. Every hour take a stand and stretch break.

5. **Miscellaneous**
   I would recommend that he/she not participate in maintenance shut downs at this time. Also, I would recommend that he avoid unplugging chutes or shoveling. He/she continues to have difficulty with these activities and it would be unsafe at this time. Also, he/she should avoid any overtime until he adjusts to an 8 hour schedule.

The above recommendations and limitations have been discussed with him/her. He/she feels that he will be able to do the chip dumping operator position with minimal difficulty. If he/she begins to have problems with the job, he will nofity his/her supervisor or medical department as soon as possible. If you should have any further questions regarding this Job Analysis, please do not hesitate to contact me.

Sincerely,

Figure 4–18.

March 20, 1988

TO: Dr. Jones

FROM: MPTC

RE: Job Analysis

The purpose of the following recommendations for his/her work site is to avoid further injury to his/her right wrist and to promote safety and well being. If you should have any questions please contact me at our Scarborough office.

I. **DESK**
The desk he/she is using at this time measures 29½". Problems which may arise from this height are neck and shoulder pain or carpal tunnel syndrome. Also, sharp edges on the desk which could increase pressure on the nerves in the forearm/elbow area.

Recommendations
A. The desk height should be 26½"–28". At this time it was discussed that we raise his/her chair 2".
B. Round the edges of the desk to decrease pressure on the forearms.

II. **CHAIR**
His/her chair height at this time is 15½" with good back support. Problems which may arise from this seat height are neck and shoulder pain.

Recommendations
A. Ergonomic Guidelines
   1. 4–5 prong base with swivel casters
   2. 10–11½" back rest adjustable 2"
   3. Seat height 16" to 22" adjustable
   4. Front edge of seat with material that breathes
   5. Seat width 15–16" allowing comfortable sitting without placing pressure behind knees.
   6. Lumbar region that tilts at less than 80–120 to give low back support.

Again, at this time it was discussed to raise his/her chair 2". Also, the seat width was increased to decrease the complaints of pressure behind the knees.

B. To avoid low back strain from prolonged sitting consider:
   1. Sit in chair with hips and knees kept at right angles, feet flat on floor.
   2. Utilize the entire seat with low back resting firmly on the back rest.
   3. A footstool maybe used to change positions to eliminate stress on low back.
   4. Change positions frequently by shifting weight or adjusting the chair.
   5. Every hour take a stand and stretch break.

The above were discussed with him/her secondary to the amount of time he/she is required to sit.

III. **GRINDING**
The grinder he/she is using is 6½" from the edge of the desk and 5" above the desk. Potential problems include wrist, neck and shoulder pain and carpal tunnel syndrome.

Recommendations
A. Push the grinder back so he/she can rest her forearm on the table and allowing her shoulders to relax.
B. Concentrate on keeping the right wrist in a neutral position to prevent further strain on the wrist. He/she was instructed to wear his/her splint if necessary to remind him/her of this position.

IV. **WIRE BENDING, PAINTING, ETC. . .**
He/She is required to use both hands for repetitive movement while using; pliers, brushes, knives, and spatulas. Potential problems include wrist, shoulder and neck pain or carpal tunnel syndrome.

Recommendations
A. Use splint when doing repetitive activities for long periods of time or when you feel the wrist fatiguing.
B. Avoid pressure over the carpal tunnel area.
C. Avoid excessive wrist movements by keeping it in a neutral position.
D. Keep the shoulders in a comfortable relaxed position.

Figure 4–19.

you know that you have some clients with this problem, you can provide more nonthreatening options to the group. Another method of control is to form teams whose participants have varied skill levels. Dynohour sounds like added work and responsibility for the provider, but social skills are a critical component to successful return to the workforce.

Stress Management

Stress management, to address the client's psychosocial needs, is also a part of every injured worker's program. The inherent stressors of the injured worker's plight include financial difficulties, family problems, spousal issues, personal issues including pain and self-esteem, frustration, inactivity, and weight gain. Thinking back to "Maslow's Hierarchy of Needs," we can see that these issues target the very core of a human being's needs for safety, shelter, food, love, and, a little further up on the scale, the need to feel good about oneself. If the baseline needs are threatened, the client cannot concentrate on rehabilitation and healing. The stress management therapist guides the client through a self-discovery process to permit him to concentrate on healing and returning to a more normal lifestyle.

How do we choose the stress management therapist who will best suit the work hardening population's needs? This can be a difficult process at best. AT MPTC, we have contracted professionals from several different disciplines, including a movement therapist, a psychologist, a psychiatrist, and a social worker (MSW) with expertise in dealing with chronic pain issues. The injured workers responded best to the MSW. This is not to say that a professional from a different discipline would not work out better for your facility. The most important attributes to look for are chronic pain expertise and a philosophy that fits the philosophy of your facility. For example, if your work hardening program emphasizes self-reliance and achievement despite adversity but the stress management therapist's emphasis is on pampering and giving in to adversity, i.e., "if you hurt stay home and do nothing," your clients will receive mixed messages. And worse yet, they will choose the message that feels most comfortable at the time. It is a scenario for failure. In interviewing for this contract position, it may help to present several potential situations and ask how the interviewee would handle the situation. The person who presents a compatible philosophy is the person to hire. The key to this, of course, is to be sure not to share too much information regarding the expected response beforehand. This usually can be accomplished best by posing this question at the beginning of the interview.

The format for stress management classes (SMCs) is usually a group format. By providing group classes, the cost for supplying this service is kept more reasonable. For the more involved client who needs individual counseling, other resources must be sought. I have not found Workers' Compensation insurance carriers to be open to taking financial responsibility for provision of these services. The cost of the group program is borne by the work hardening facility. When calculating the charge for work hardening services, any contract providers' salaries should be included in the expenses column.

Group classes held twice a week have worked well at our center. We also have tried one longer session that is 90 minutes rather than two 45-minute sessions, but we found it to be too overwhelming for most clients to handle. The client's comfort level is pivotal to his success in this arena. We try to schedule the client's day so that this session is a part of the time he is scheduled to be here anyway.

One of the most challenging aspects of providing SMC is to sustain the integrity of the present group while accepting new participants as they enter the work hardening program. A closed format of particular topics taught a particular way, in a particular order, has the potential to exclude some clients from class because new clients can only enter when the cycle is complete. If the cycle is shorter than the number of weeks the client is participating in the work hardening program, he is left without support for the remaining time. The most practical approach is to establish set topics to be addressed during SMC but to be flexible enough to meet the needs of the population at that time. The ultimate goal of stress management is to teach the client to become self-sufficient in coping with his stressors after work hardening is complete. Some employers have requested that their workers be allowed to attend class and/or to see the treating therapist once per week for one month after return to work to facilitate a smoother transition for the worker. If the employer is that conscientious, we try to accommodate the request.

Stress management topics that have been chosen at our facility have been identification of acceptable levels of discomfort, differentiating between "OK" pain and "not OK" pain, assertive communication skills, and coping mechanisms including relaxation techniques, physical responses to stress, and interpersonal relationships. As long as these topics are covered well enough to meet the needs of the clients, the order in which they are presented is irrelevant.

These sessions must be closed sessions that do not include family, work hardening therapists, or any other "outside" people. The issue of total privacy and the opportunity to openly discuss problems and solutions in a nonjudgmental environment is key to this program's success. Therefore, there should be a thorough understanding between the provider of SMC and the providers of work hardening regarding what approach is expected. In other words, the end goals should be compatible. The combination of a stress management provider who takes a soft line approach ("the poor baby" approach), and a work hardening provider who takes a firm approach that promotes early self-reliance, is a recipe for failure for the clients. Both parties must emphasize the injured worker's remaining function and de-emphasize the role that pain and discomfort play in the client's life. The client's remaining functional capabilities are the base skills upon which the work hardening provider stimulates the client to rebuild. The more positive approach of looking at what is remaining rather than concentrating on what was lost provides the client with a successful atmosphere in which to improve. The SMC provider also must grasp this philosophy.

A room separated from the work hardening center is provided for SMC. It should be large enough and warm enough for the clients to lay down to practice relaxation techniques. The room should be in an area free from distractions including the telephone. If an all-purpose room is used and a telephone is present, the ringer and paging system are turned off when SMCs are in session. The clients know that this is their time to vent frustrations and find solutions in a quiet, safe environment, totally uninterrupted by the world outside.

Nutrition Counseling

The final component of the work hardening program is nutrition counseling. If you have observed a problem such as abdominal obesity in a back-injured client, a medical case can be made for the necessity of weight loss to promote improvement. It is also a self-esteem issue with the client who expresses frustration regarding weight gain since the inactivity of the injury has occurred. Weight gain is cause for concern in many areas, especially cardiovascular and flexibility. The client experiencing weight gain frequently does not have clothing that fits and cannot afford new clothes. Proper stretching positions are inhibited. Social skills suffer as the embarrassed client tends not to interact.

The many ramifications of weight gain can be addressed by a registered dietician. The dietician who provides services to our clients has a private space in which she counsels the clients individually during the weekly weigh-in. Here, the dietician and client discuss any problems that have arisen over the last week and the weigh-in takes place. This individual approach appears to be more comfortable for the clients than group meetings on the very personal matter of weight control.

Behavior modification takes place as the client learns that sensible eating does not mean starvation or deprivation of all the foods the client likes to eat. Weight loss can be difficult at a time in the injured worker's life when life's pleasures seem to have dwindled to the pleasure of eating foods that he likes.

We are fortunate that the dietician who works with our clients does all of the reimbursement legwork and obtains insurance approval to provide services. We do not contract her services so there is no increased financial outlay for our facility. Nevertheless, our injured workers receive top-quality, caring counseling from this reputable company.

The need for nutritional counseling is often a difficult subject to broach. Whether it is brought up out of a concern to lose or gain weight does not appear to matter. People who are underweight can be just as offended as those who are overweight. There is no proven method of conveying this message without the client taking offense. However, the client usually receives the information well if it is presented in a caring manner and if the client's dignity is preserved. If the client himself brings up the topic of weight gain, this is the perfect opportunity to present your case for nutrition counseling. The weekly sessions should be scheduled at a time when the client is already planning to be at the work hardening center. The more convenient the appointment, the more likely it is that the client will follow through. Besides, we do not want to add to the already burdensome list of appointments that disrupt the client's life. Nutrition counseling should become something that the client does for himself, and that is also how we present work hardening. Up until now, many of the appointments that the injured worker has been forced to keep were to fulfill his obligations to his employer and the Workers' Compensation carrier. However, with the introduction of work hardening, the focus shifts to the individual taking care of himself and achieving his own personal and career goals that will permit him to return to a more normal lifestyle.

In summary, work hardening programs may include:

1. Punching a time clock
2. Independent clipboard program
3. Stretching
4. Cardiovascular activities
5. Body mechanics education
6. Job-task simulation
7. Normal workday breaks
8. Productivity circuits
9. Dynamic activity hour
10. Stress management classes
11. Nutrition counseling

During day one of work hardening, it is rare for the client to begin more than the stretching routine. The primary emphasis on this day is for the client to develop a comfort level with and an understanding of what role the work hardening program will play in his rehabilitation. By day two, the client is ready to fully participate in his work hardening program. The treating therapist should plan to spend increased time with the new client

for at least these two days. After that, the injured worker has a better understanding of the flow of the program and his responsibilities during the day.

As you can see by the sample schedules (Figures 4–20 and 4–21), the two-hour block of time in these first few days leaves virtually no time for specific job tasks other than those incorporated into the body mechanics part.

Daily Schedule

Date	4-6	4-7	4-8	4-9	4-10	4-13	4-14	4-15	4-16
Hours	2 hrs.	2 hrs.	2 hrs.	2 hrs.	2 hrs.	4 hrs.	2 hrs.	4 hrs.	2 hrs.
Upper Body Warm-Up *	orientation	10x	10x	10x	10x	10x	10x	10x	10x
Lower Body Warm-Up	orientation	10x	10x	10x	10x	10x	10x	10x	10x
Back Exercises	screening	stress mgmt.	10x	10x	stress mgmt.	10x	stress mgmt.	10x	15x •
Treadmill	screening	stress mgmt.	Dyno hr.	5 min.	stress mgmt.	7 min. •	stress mgmt.	Dyno hr.	7 min.
Lower Extremity Exercises	screening		Dyno hr.	10x	back ex. 10x	10x (break)	back ex. 10x	(break)	10x
Circuit I						45 min.		45 min.	
Upper Extremity Exercises						10x		10x	
Ergonomic Bike						5 min.		5 min.	
Cool Downs ✓						5x		5x	

Name_____ Ben D. Nees _____

Figure 4–20. Daily Schedule Flow Chart for Back Injured Clients Work Hardening Tasks

Daily Schedule

Date	8-1	8-2	8-3	8-4	8-5	8-8	8-9	8-10	8-11
Hours	2 hrs.	2 hrs.	2 hrs.	2 hrs.	2 hrs.	2 hrs.	2 hrs.	2 hrs.	2 hrs.
Upper Body Warm-Up *	NMSS	10x	10x	10x	10x	10x	10x	10x	10x
Theraband	NMSS	10x yellow	10x	10x	10x	10x	10x	10x red	10x
Lower Body Exercises	orien- tation	stress mgmt. 45 min.	10x	10x	stress mgmt. 45 min.	10x	stress mgmt. 45 min.	10x	10x
Ergonomic Bike (push/pull only)	orien- tation	5 min.	5 min.	7 min. •	stress mgmt. 45 min.	7 min.	7 min.	8 min. •	8 min.
Upper Extremity Exercises	orien- tation	cage levels 5-6-7	Dyno hr.	10x	cage levels 5-6-7	10x wts. added, see 5-6-7 ex's •	cage levels	10x	10x
		no cage done due to heat		CA					

Name_____ Carrie Proppa _____

Figure 4–21.   Daily Schedule Flow Chart for Upper Extremity Injured Clients Work Hardening Tasks

CHAPTER 5

Advancing the Client's Program

Let us assume that the client has been in the work hardening program for a few nondescript days. How do we know when to advance the client and in which areas? The changes the treating therapist will see tend to be more subtle than the changes observed in the acute care clinic. For example, has the client experienced signs and symptoms of flare-up, e.g., redness, swelling, heat, sensory changes, circulatory changes, or discomfort? Have control mechanisms kept these flare-ups contained to a reasonable level? If not, then the client is not ready to advance. If the changes are contained, then progress in the more subtle form of increased repetitions or an added activity may be fine. However, we would not increase several activities in the program at one time. It is important to note which activities are tolerated best. This is better accomplished in the more fragile work hardening client by advancing the program in a more step-wise fashion. If the client has not experienced any negative reactions to his increased activity level, then he is ready for more challenge. With the many facets of the program, the client's progress can take multiple forms, including repetitions, resistance, and improved heart rate, body mechanics, independence, and productivity, as well as increased time in the program.

The next aspect to consider is the use of modalities, such as heat, ice, or transcutaneous electrical nerve stimulation (TENS). Because work hardening is a program that should be initiated only after addressing the acute phase of injury, generally modalities are not an accepted part of the client's workday. In some programs, heat and ice are permitted as long as the client identifies the need for them. Demonstrations of exaggerated pain behaviors are not tolerated nor are they acknowledged by treating personnel. For instance, if a client moans, grunts, rubs, limps, shakes a body part, or grimaces, the treating therapist will not offer an ice massage. Manipulative behaviors are not reinforced. However, if that client approaches the treating therapist and states that an ice massage would be helpful to alleviate increased symptoms, he will receive an ice massage.

Progress in the use of modalities is measured in several ways. Does the client still need heat prior to beginning his program or does he wait until half way through or until the end? Does he still require heat or ice every day? Is he wearing the TENS unit when he arrives or does he wait until part way through the program? Does he still require a modality at home to sleep at night? Is the modality used in conjunction with pain medication or has he been able to stop taking the medication? Improvement in any of these areas means progress.

Is the injured worker compliant with his program? If he does not arrive on time, skips days, does not complete all activities, refuses to take seriously the body mechanics instructions, or changes parts of the program without permission, this client cannot safely progress. If attendance is poor at two hours daily, it will not improve by increasing to four hours per day. The injured worker must follow the rules and regulations of the work hardening program before increasing his responsibilities beyond the base level.

Another component to consider in expanding the client's program is his readiness for home carryover. All clients need to supplement the center's program with carryover at home. This reinforcement during the missed days assures more consistent performance of daily tasks. It also returns some of the control for the injured worker's recovery back to his hands. Instilling this responsibility early in the program gives the client plenty of time to adjust for when he is no longer involved in the work hardening program. The most critical element used to determine readiness for home carryover is the client's demonstration of good technique during the observed time spent in the return-to-work center. As the client's techniques improve, he can be assigned a home program with confidence that he will perform the tasks safely. Assignment of a home program constitutes progress.

The client will not necessarily know the philosophy behind the layout of his program, but he must be provided with enough information to be comfortable with the "why's" of his program. For example, if he knows that carrying a bucket 10 feet will eventually lead to carrying his load at work for 50 feet, he is much more likely to participate fully. The client must be kept abreast of the end-point goals so that he can relate what he is doing to what he has to do at work. His willingness to continue may be contingent on this information, especially if the client wants to be fully rehabilitated yesterday. This client is overly motivated and needs a full explanation of the tasks in his program so that he does not overdo and reinjure. It is very difficult for such clients to take rehabilitation in stride. However, when furnished with enough information to draw their own conclusions, a full understanding of the work hardening program develops. Demonstrated understanding of the program is considered progress. Once this occurs, the client's program can be increased in weights, repetitions, length of day, time spent in cardiovascular training, and introduction of productivity circuits.

MEASURING PROGRESS

Progress is measured both physically and psychosocially. Psychological readiness to advance may be more difficult to assess. To determine this, take your cues from the client's body language and from what he says to coworkers and to the treating therapists. The client's general attitude is displayed clearly during the FCA and work hardening orientation session. If he is cooperative, motivated, anxious, depressed, skeptical, or angry, you will know it. In the work hardening program, try to keep the motivated clients challenged and to see a positive change in the less cooperative client's attitude. Sometimes, a positive change occurs just because the work atmosphere of the work hardening center is familiar ground. In other words, the client strongly identifies with his working role in society. The original negativity was from the frustration of being excluded from this role and feeling useless. Of course, not all clients respond strictly because of the surroundings of the work center and, therefore, they may need more direct input to make progress. Because the injured worker spends so much time with you in an informal, group atmosphere, getting to know the little nuances of what is important to him is usually a matter of making the effort to spend some time with him while he executes his assigned program. Through this approach, the client also learns that he can trust you. He will "open up" and his psychological readiness to progress should become apparent. Here are some techniques to assist clients with developing a comfort level with a therapist:

1. When speaking with a client, go to his level. If he is working on the floor, sit on the floor beside him. Hovering over someone is a power position. It makes the uncomfortable client feel inferior and resentful.

2. Speak the client's language. Listen to the words he uses to determine if he uses more words that refer to feeling or touch, hearing, tasting, smelling, or seeing. He will respond better when spoken to in his dominant style. For example, "that sounds right to me" or "I see what you mean."

3. Always correct the client's technique on a personal level. It can be done quietly while the client is attempting the task. I have been present in some facilities when corrections have been indiscriminately screamed across the room. How embarrassing for the client!

4. If during the course of conversation a personal issue arises, offer to take the client to a private area, as emotions are frequently more fragile during this time. If the client breaks down and cries, he will be less embarrassed if the therapist is the only other person present. The client's dignity remains intact.

5. Take a firm stand on issues that affect client success. For example, if a client complains of discomfort from the work hardening program, charge him with identifying which activity it is that causes the problem. It is not the whole program. Once the problem task is identified, find a different method of performing that task to better fit the client's present needs.

6. Provide the client with a full explanation of the particular setup of his program. He may need to know why his program is different from someone else's. An explanation will map out the methodology leading from his work hardening activities to accomplishment of his goals. It gives the client a reason to trust you.

7. Take the time to point out the client's successes. They are oftentimes very subtle and undetected by the client. A success could be something as simple as lifting correctly one time out of five attempts. The injured worker frequently has been programmed to fail long before he enters work hardening. As he relearns the feeling of success, his motivation and self-esteem improve.

There are many other techniques, but the above points are some of the most important issues to be addressed. These points are emphasized because these are the ones most quickly forgotten or never learned. With a field as new as work hardening, most of us are not privileged with a mentor who can coach us and give us the answers. Some of the interpersonal skills needed by treating therapists do not come naturally and must be learned. And on the opposite end of the scale are those of us who become a little "battle hardened" through the years and need a reminder of the subtle components, the humanitarian elements of what we bring to the work hardening center. Indeed, it is these elements that help our most needy clients to achieve success.

The issue of trust is always important in any human relationship. Unfortunately, there can be a fine line between the client trusting the treating therapist and crossing over into total dependence on the therapist and the program. Initially, having lost so much control over his life, the client may have difficulty assuming responsibility for his own life again. Signs of this dependence oftentimes show up when return to work is imminent. When the therapist recognizes that this is a problem, the client must be handled with care. Time should be spent reinforcing the gains that the client has made and crediting his efforts with this success. Many clients say "I don't know what I would have done without you and this program." This grateful comment is always received openly with an addendum statement from the therapist such as "you would not be where you are without your dedication and commitment to the program." Once this comment is made, an effort is made to constantly barrage the client with positive reinforcers that indicate that he will be fine without work hardening because he is now ready to care for himself. This message is already a part of the work hardening protocol, but some clients have a more difficult time integrating that concept than others.

CLIPBOARD PROGRAM

Now that we are prepared to assess the client's readiness to advance in the program, a further explanation of the clipboard program is in order. On the client's clipboard are a daily schedule sheet, exercise instruction sheets, and a circuit sheet. The client should be able to carry out his day's tasks independently with these documents. All sheets on the clipboard program have the client's name on them to prevent mix-up of programs once several clients are participating at the same time. The clients take their programs apart and leave them scattered in different areas of the center. Placing the names on the pages decreases the likelihood that John will inherit Mary's activities sheets.

Daily Schedule

The daily schedule pages, samples of which are in *Appendix A*, have a complete listing of the tasks to be achieved that day. At the top of the document is the day's date and the number of hours the client will be attending. With many programs to write, this information is helpful in determining the list of tasks for the next day without having to pull the client's chart. The schedule is written daily after assessing the client's response to the present day's activities. Because there is no way to know the client's response in advance, the schedule cannot be written several days at a time. If the client is not responding well, the daily schedule may not increase. However, because this is part of the client's record, a new column should be written with a new date every day. This also assures that the program is reviewed daily.

The idea of the clipboard program is to facilitate independence. However, if the therapist does not put enough information on the daily schedule, the injured worker still will need to check back constantly with the therapist. Insufficient information undermines the purpose of the setup. Use symbols next to the activity name that corresponds to the symbol on another sheet. For example, if you use stars next to the exercises you want the client to do during the warm-up period, also put a star next to the task on the daily schedule sheet (Figure 4–22). Color coding works well to draw attention to changes in an activity or as cuing for the client who does not read well. Also be sure to include the number of repetitions, amount of weight or resistance, distance to be travelled, height levels, time to be spent, and rest periods to be taken.

Be as specific as possible without being overly verbose and confusing. Besides providing the client with all of the information necessary to carry out his program independently, the therapist has a permanent record of that client's activities. For example, if a case should ever go to court, testimony may not be called for until a year or more after you have treated the client. The more complete the record, the easier it is to give testimony accurately.

Exercises

The daily schedule pages also list exercises, such as upper body warm-ups, upper extremity exercises, lower body exercises, and cool-downs. Such exercises are used to provide the more muscle-specific aspects of the beginning work hardening program. Approximately 70 such exercises are shown in *Appendix B*, grouped according to body area. The asterisks and check marks found on some of the exercise sheets correspond to those found on the daily schedule forms.

Each of the exercises has a space for the length of time to hold a muscle contraction, and for the number of repetitions of a movement. Both time and number should be determined by a therapist on an individual basis.

In acute care therapy, a program such as this would be prohibitively time-consuming. However, because work hardening clients spend from two to eight hours per day in the program, a comprehensive warm-up, strengthening, and cool-down is frequently necessary.

Circuit Sheet

The other component of the client's clipboard program that may require further explanation is the circuit sheet. The date and the number of hours the client is to be present on that day is recorded as it is on the daily schedule. The circuit is an activity that would be listed on the daily schedule. The word "circuit" usually is written in the activities column on the daily schedule with the amount of time to be spent on that circuit written in the specific day column. The circuit sheet is comprised of a list of job-specific tasks (Figures 5–1 and 5–2). Circuits rarely are added to the client's program until he is ready to spend four hours or more in the work hardening center. Clients participate in two-hour blocks of time—two, four, six, and eight hours. Although the emphasis in work hardening is on return to work, the reality is that the client has to return to life. Therefore, some of the activities in which the client participates also will enhance life skills. However, the circuit's primary goals are strictly work-oriented, as they represent the client's job dissected into its smallest components. Other activities will be listed on the daily schedule. Circuits are concentrated efforts to address feasibility issues. This is where the client and therapist problem solve regarding work-related issues such as pacing, work technique, and alternative work methods. It is the arena in which the client is provided the opportunity to recover to pre-injury levels and to demonstrate his improvement to himself and to the medical community who will release him back to the workforce.

The list of activities on the circuit sheets should be kept to a maximum of four to five tasks. This permits more accurate assessment of the results. If the client's job is so complex that it can be broken down into 10 tasks, for example, begin with five of those tasks on one circuit and wait a few days to assess the results. A second circuit can be added when the first group of tasks is under control. It is not unusual to have a client performing more than one circuit.

The specificity required of the daily schedule also is required of the circuit. Codes and symbols likewise can be used to enhance the client's understanding. Although our therapists do not move the circuits to the next column every day, as in the daily schedule, the circuits are reviewed daily for potential changes. The primary reason for not rewriting them is to save on time spent doing paperwork. When the client's daily schedule is reviewed, the circuit is addressed. Therefore, there is a built-in check to be sure the review is completed.

EVENTS LEADING TO DISCHARGE

To this point we have addressed initiating and advancing the client's program. So how do we know when to discharge the client? Most work hardening programs run from four to six weeks. We have noted at MPTC that back-injured clients generally work through the program at a quicker pace than upper-extremity–injured clients. As a general population, the clients with upper-extremity injuries enter the program with more psychological overlay. It would be interesting to see a study published on this phenomenon. Not all clients jump from two- to four- to six- to eight-hour days five days per week, either. Some clients need to alternate days when increasing; for example, three four-hour days and two six-hour days. The length of the program in weeks will be dependent on the needs of the client, but your facility should make a policy as to the maximum acceptable number. You also should know if your Workers' Compensation system has established parameters already.

When the client's progress has stopped or slowed to an imperceptible level, he should be discharged. What if he has not reached work-level parameters? If this is the case, the therapist can recommend return to work at the established level. The client will continue a program at home or at a local health club. Although the out-of-work issue is resolved, the client may want to continue to try to make gains, however slow, to regain his prior job in the company. There are many companies who reward this effort by paying for YMCA or health club memberships.

A second reason for discharge is that goals have been reached: a full, 40-hour workweek is demonstrated, body mechanics are ingrained, pain is under control, and work feasibility issues have been resolved.

Finally, discharge also may take place due to noncompliance with the program. Noncompliance takes many forms. Among them are, erratic attendance; alcohol or drug abuse, or both; poor attitude; and unsafe practices. Most of these points are self-explanatory. Poor attitude may appear to be a judgment call that is difficult to back up, but good documentation prior to discharge should support the therapist's decision. A client with a bitter, negative attitude unresolved through stress management counseling can taint the entire group of work hardening participants when he is there. This is unacceptable. Besides the repercussions in the work hardening population, the client himself will not improve.

With the client's discharge planned, what have the treating professionals learned about this client's return-to-work capabilities? The physician who signs the return-to-work order will look for direction regarding

Date	8/12	8/15	8/16	8/17	8/18	8/19	8/22	8/23	8/24
Hours	4 hrs.	4 hrs.	4 hrs.	4 hrs.	4 hrs.	6 hrs.	6 hrs.	4 hrs.	6 hrs.
Flip Switch (alternate arms)	1 min.	1 min.	1 1/2 min.●	1 1/2 min.	2 min. ●	2 min.	2 min.	2 min.	2 1/2 min. ●
Push Button	5x	5x	5x	5x	5x	5x	5x	5x	5x
List Numbers	1 row	1 row	1 row	1 row	1 row	1 row	1 row	1 row	1 row
Carry Crate	11#	11#	15# ●	15#	20# ●	20#	23# ●	23#	23#
						CA			

Name **Carrie Proppa**

Figure 5–1. Circuit Included in Daily Schedule for Upper Extremity Injured Client

Date	8/25	8/26	8/29	9/1	9/2	9/5	9/6	9/7	9/8
Hours	6 hrs.	6 hrs.	6 hrs.	8 hrs.	8 hrs.	8 hrs.	8 hrs.	8 hrs.	8 hrs.
Flip Switch (alternate arms)	2 1/2 min.	2 1/2 min.	3 min.•	3 min.	3 min.	3 1/2 • min.	3 1/2 min.	3 1/2 min.	3 1/2 min.
Push Button	5x	5x	5x	5x	5x	5x	5x	5x	5x
List Numbers	1 row	1 row	1 row	2 rows•	2 rows	2 rows	2 rows	2 rows	2 rows
Carry Crate	25# •	25#	25# •	27# •	27# •	27#	30# •	30#	30#
						CA			

Name _____ Carrie Proppa _____

Figure 5–1. (continued)

Circuit

Date	8/19	8/22	8/24	8/25	8/26	8/29	9/1	9/2	9/5
Hours	6 hrs.	6 hrs.	6 hrs.	6 hrs.	6 hrs.	6 hrs.	8 hrs.	8 hrs.	8 hrs.
Minnesota (Alt. sit/ stand)	flip 1 side	flip 1 side	flip 1 side	flip 1 side	flip 1 side	flip 1 side	flip 1 side	flip 1 side	flip 1 side
String	10x around ea. set● (3)	10x around	10x around	20x around●	20x around	20x around	20x around	20x around	20x around
Cage (levels off & on)	5-6-7	5-6-7	5-6-7	5-6-7	5-6-7	5-6-7	5-6-7	5-6-7	5-6-7

Name_____Carrie Proppa_____

Figure 5–2. Continuation of Second Circuit for Upper Extremity Injured Client

Date	9/6	9/7	9/8						
Hours	6 hrs.	6 hrs.	6 hrs.						
Minnesota (Alt. sit/ stand)	flip 1 side	flip 1 side	flip 1 side						
String	20x around	20x around	20x around						
Crawford 90° work surface (sit or stand)	2 rows each	2 rows each	2 rows each						
Cage (levels off & on)	5-6-7	5-6-7	5-6-7						

Name_____Carrie Proppa_____

Figure 5–2. (continued)

return-to-work recommendations. During the work hardening program, the client demonstrates increasing work capabilities during job simulation. He gradually increases the level of difficulty and the hours spent performing these tasks. But sometimes, the client's capabilities in a certain area are not clear. If this is the case, a final FCA should be done. Maybe it does not need to be as comprehensive as the original evaluation, as cost is always a consideration. But a shortened version covering the unclear points will be helpful. The final FCA also presents the opportunity to compare original parameters with final parameters. Depending on the reason for the work hardening program, a final FCA could be a waste of money. Each case must be judged on its own merit. A client who during work hardening clearly demonstrates the capabilities necessary to return to his job does not need a final assessment.

If a job analysis has not been performed and the information needed to make appropriate recommendations for return to work is incomplete, a last-ditch effort should be made to obtain permission to go to the jobsite and obtain the necessary data. Some employers are reluctant to have you perform an ergonomic job analysis and you cannot get them to agree to it. Some employers are defense contractors or have company secrets regarding equipment design and need reassurance of our professionalism and trustworthiness. In these cases, I agree to videotape the job and then stay onsite to evaluate the tape and dictate my report. When I leave the plant, the videotape stays with them. I charge more for this service because I am unavailable to my company during this time. The employer also must provide a room for me to work in and the viewing equipment necessary. However, this compromise resolves the secrecy issues satisfactorily while providing me with the information necessary to make an appropriate recommendation. If the treating therapist is uncertain about any phase of the client's job, the recommendation at the completion of work hardening is that the client can return to work to his previous job if his final work hardening capabilities match those required to safely perform the job. However, if the therapist knows the client's job tasks, the recommendations for return to work can be much more specific.

You may be questioning how we initiate true work hardening without a job analysis. The answer is, with great difficulty. However, with the client's information provided on the job questionnaire and a good job description that is not disputed by the client, work hardening can take place. Nevertheless, when discharge time arrives, the recommendation to return to work is qualified as follows:

I recommend return to work at full duty if the written information provided to me by the company is accurate. If the information is questionable, I recommend that the client work within the parameters established during his work hardening program. An ergonomic job analysis would clarify all points. However, the employer has denied access to MPTC to perform a proper job analysis.

If the physician feels uncomfortable with the lack of cooperation by the employer, he may not sign the return-to-work order until a full job analysis is allowed.

On occasion, there will be a lag time between when the client is discharged and return to the job. When this occurs, there is always the danger that the client will lose ground. To prevent this from happening, contact the Workers' Compensation carrier to request weekly visits for a specified period of time. During the weekly visit, the client is re-evaluated by having him perform his complete program just the same as at the time of discharge. If home carryover has been poor, the client will have difficulty with this weekly visit. If this turns out to be the case, closer supervision is recommended. The insurance carrier is usually very cooperative regarding increasing the client's visits to two or three times per week until the client demonstrates more consistent home carryover. If he finds he has to return more frequently, the client quickly recognizes that shirking his responsibilities to maintain the capabilities gained during the work hardening leads to more regimented supervision. Nonetheless, an end point must be established for the length of time your facility is willing to do this and for how long the insurance company believes this approach is feasible. With this procedure, you also could be accused of babysitting. It does not work for everybody. But for those clients who initially have difficulty with self-discipline, this approach is a great success. Also, most of your clients will not require this follow-up treatment because they have been ingrained with the concept of independence right from the beginning with the early initiation of their home program.

At discharge, a graduation of sorts takes place. After all, this is an accomplishment that demanded the client's full cooperation and participation. The success is to his credit and we celebrate that with him by presenting to him a graduation certificate hailing his accomplishment. The entire group participates in the celebration of success during morning break. It is a positive experience for the whole group. The clients become closely knit during their weeks together and begin to identify with each other's failures and successes. So, if we have the opportunity to encourage the clients through their co-worker's success, we take full advantage of it.

Finally, a discharge letter is prepared. This letter is sent to all involved professionals. It can be designed as a form letter so that the therapists can just fill in the blanks. Another nice feature of a form letter, besides the convenience, is that it functions as a reminder of which information needs to be included. Among the points that should be included are:

1. Length of time in the program, giving dates.
2. Number of sessions scheduled and sessions attended.
3. Consistency of attendance.
4. Final functional capabilities.
5. Return-to-work recommendations.
6. Areas of improvement observed during work hardening.

Copies of this discharge letter may go to the physician, rehabilitation/vocational counselor, Workers' Compensation insurance carrier, attorney, and employer.

The discharge letter should bring to light all of the client's gains including the less obvious ones. Once a client completed the program, I performed a final FCA, and the resistances demonstrated had not improved significantly. I was shocked to think that, although the client's endurance had improved enough for her to safely return to the workforce, her lifting, carrying, pushing, and pulling were just slightly better than at the initial FCA. After giving myself a day to distance myself from the emotional aspect of the situation, I sat down and re-evaluated the results. In fact, the client had made many improvements. She demonstrated no pain behaviors throughout the assessment. She described pain that was minimal and much less severe than it was originally. Her body mechanics were impeccable. Durations and frequency had improved. Indeed, she was a much more feasible employee than the one who entered the work hardening program.

Use your observation skills to their fullest when reviewing final work parameters. Expect the unexpected. Results and improvements vary considerably from client to client. In the example above, I expected to see big gains in resistances, but instead found big gains elsewhere, and that was all right. The client successfully returned to the workforce.

CHAPTER 6

Documentation

Documentation in work hardening involves more paperwork than in an acute care clinic. The additional charting comes from the revision of the client's clipboard program every day. Although the look of the work hardening program paperwork might not be exactly the same in all work hardening facilities, the general flavor is the same.

The "to do's" of documenting include:

1. Put the dates of service on all documents.
2. Put the client's name on all documents.
3. Document all cancellations and no-shows.
4. Document the date of the next physician appointment.
5. Be clear and complete—over- rather than under-document.

The reason for being so picky is for future reference. Dates and names on all documents save a lot of time later on. One timesaver we use is a mini-monthly attendance record placed at the top of the progress notes so we can see at a glance consistency of attendance (Figure 6–1). This is especially helpful when receiving a telephone call, for instance, from a rehabilitation counselor with a question. We do not delay them on the telephone while leafing through paperwork to provide information regarding attendance. We gain credibility also when providing quick information.

Daily Progress Notes

Daily progress notes can be written in a narrative or subjective, objective, assessment, and plans (SOAP) format, whatever your facility is most comfortable with. The therapist or licensed assistant can write these notes (check with your own state regulations regarding this). The daily notes include:

1. Whether the client completed the program
2. Pain reports
3. Pain behaviors
4. Psychosocial complaints
5. Whether progress was made

6. Modalities received, when, and what kind
7. Private meetings held, with whom, and why
8. Classes attended
9. Job analysis attended
10. Meetings with involved professionals
11. Derogatory remarks
12. Plans for next day
13. Correspondence sent on client's behalf
14. Cancellations and reason, no-shows, and attempts to reach client
15. Client's name and the date

Weekly Progress Note

The weekly progress note replaces the daily notes. At our facility, it is always the therapist who is responsible for completing this. It includes everything that is included in a daily note only in weekly form. It summarizes what has occurred over the last week and the goals planned for the following week. To assist with this process, weekly interdisciplinary meetings are held. In facilities where there are contract people involved, not everyone will attend this meeting. Because of this, it is important to obtain feedback from contract personnel while they are at the facility.

The Daily Schedule Sheet

Although the daily schedule sheet (Figure 6–2) already has been introduced in chapter 5, a list of its components is included here to have all documentation in one section. The daily schedule sheet is the client's list of activities to be completed for that day. It includes:

1. Date and number of hours in attendance
2. Changes in assigned activities
3. Classes to be attended
4. Cancellations and no-shows
5. Professional meetings
6. Color coding and symbols to enhance understanding
7. List of activities, heights, weights, resistances, times, and repetitions.

Month	Yr	1	2	3	4	5	6	7	8	9	10	11	12	13	14	15	16	17	18	19	20	21	22	23	24	25	26	27	28	29	30	31

DATE	PROGRESS NOTES

Figure 6–1. Sample Progress Notes Sheet with Three Month Grid to Provide At-A-Glance Attendance Record

Daily Schedule

Date									
Hours									

Name_____

Figure 6–2. Blank Daily Schedule Form for Reader's Use in their Facility

8. Target heart rate
9. Client's name

The daily schedule sheet is intended to facilitate the client's independence in assuming responsibility for his own rehabilitation. Therefore, the more information we can provide in a concise manner, the better it is for the client.

Also, the insurance companies frequently request copies of the injured worker's program and notes. By providing many days' worth of activities on one sheet of paper, it becomes more readable for the claims adjuster and less costly to photocopy.

The daily schedule sheet is reviewed and rewritten in the next column every day. In the column of activities, cancellations and no-shows are documented in red pen so that they are clearly visible.

The Circuit Sheet

Again, this document already has been introduced, but it is beneficial to have it here as well (Figure 6–3). The circuit sheet is a list of work-related tasks that the client performs for a specified period of time or for a specified number of repetitions, depending on what the circuit is meant to accomplish. For example, if the client works too fast and does not pace well, the circuit can be used to document number of tasks per unit of time. The circuit sheet includes:

1. Date and number of hours in attendance
2. Client's name
3. List of assigned tasks including heights, weights, resistances, distances, repetitions, and time.
4. Color coding and other symbols
5. Changes in assigned activities

The circuit sheet activities, although reviewed every day, are not rewritten in the next column until there is a change in the activities. Because the daily schedule is moved to a new column every day, the circuit, which is one of the daily schedule activities, is tracked there.

Progress Letter to Physician

A letter regarding the client's progress always is sent with the client when he is scheduled to see the physician (Figure 6–4). Although some of our clients still are seeing their physicians every one to two weeks, this letter provides an objective outline of the client's progress. The physician does not have to rely on the client's accuracy

and reporting skills. It also provides the therapist with the opportunity to obtain the physician's feedback on a consistent basis regarding suggested future plans for the client. The progress letter fosters the teamwork necessary to provide a successful work hardening program.

The progress letter includes:

1. Usual letter heading and date
2. Client's name
3. Length of time client has been in program
4. Number of scheduled sessions versus number attended
5. Consistency of attendance
6. Number of hours per session in the beginning and now
7. Progress made in strength, endurance, pain control, function, and attendance
8. Modalities
9. Classes attended
10. Plans regarding further treatment

If this is set up as a form letter, it is easy to fill out in a short time period. Our clients carry their progress letters in open envelopes. Frequently we review what we have put inside if there is any question that the client may not be able to read it and understand it himself. If the client ever fails to give the note to the physician, any future letters are mailed directly to the physician. As with all documents, a copy is placed into the client's permanent record. If you also have agreed to keep the insurance carrier and/or rehabilitation counselor up-to-date in writing, a copy of the physician's letter suffices nicely.

Discharge

As stated in the previous chapter, the discharge letter and discharge summary (Figures 6–5 and 6–6) are the final steps in the discharge process. They include:

1. Length of time in program, giving dates
2. Number of sessions scheduled and attended
3. Consistency of attendance
4. Final functional parameters
5. Return-to-work recommendations
6. Areas of improvement

It is like any other correspondence sent to the physician. The facts should be stated with follow-up and return-to-work recommendations.

Circuit

Date									
Hours									

Name_____

Figure 6–3. Blank Circuit Form for Reader's Use in their Facility

PHYSICIAN'S PROGRESS LETTER SAMPLE

Date

M.D.
M.D. Place
City, State Zip Code

Dear M.D.:

Mr./Mrs./Ms. _____**name**_____ has been attending Work Hardening since _____**date**_____.
He/She has attended _____**#**_____ out of _____**#**_____ scheduled treatment sessions. (Note here if consistency has been a problem.) He/She began the daily program for _____**#**_____ hours per day and has increased to/remained at _____**#**_____ hours. He/She is progressing with respect to (strength, endurance, function, etc.) Mr./Mrs./Ms. _____**name**_____ requires a hot pack (other modalities) half way through the session and notes relief from **discomfort, spasm, etc.** He/She is attending Stress Management and appears to benefit via improved coping skills.

We plan to continue the client in this program for _____**time**_____ working towards
Mr./Mrs./Ms. _____**name**_____ goals. If you have any questions or concerns, please contact me.

Sincerely,

Figure 6–4. Sample of Physician's Progress Letter in present Format to be used in Reader's Clinic for Work Hardening Progress Letter to Physicians.

DISCHARGE SUMMARY

Name: _____ Date of Evaluation: _____

Diagnosis: _____ Date of Discharge: _____

Doctor: _____ Number of Visits: _____

Condition when initially seen: _____

_____

_____

Summary of treatment:_____

_____

_____

Condition at time of discharge:_____

_____

_____

Comments/Recommendations:_____

_____

_____

Unless I am contacted by your office, I will consider this patient to be discharged from physical therapy at this time. If you have any further questions or concerns, please feel free to contact me at our Scarborough/Saco/Biddeford office.

_____

Figure 6–5. Sample Blank Discharge Summary for Reader's Use in their Facility

DISCHARGE SUMMARY

Name: _____ Date of Evaluation: February 5, 1991

Diagnosis: R shld/L hip tendonitis _____ Date of Discharge: March 29, 1991

Doctor: _____ Number of Visits: 25 out of 27 scheduled

Condition when initially seen: Generalized upper body discomfort right greater than left, four hour workday

tolerance, unable to perform work tasks.

Summary of treatment: Attended Work Hardening progressing from two hours to eight hours five days per

week, attended consistently, work simulated tasks performed.

Condition at time of discharge: Eight hour work day tolerance, parameters as per Functinoal Capacity

Assessment performed March 27, 1991. Body Mechanics and Posture improved.

Comments/Recommendations: return to work as per Functional Capacity Assessment

Unless I am contacted by your office, I will consider this patient to be discharged from physical therapy at this time. If you have any further questions or concerns, please feel free to contact me at our Scarborough/Saco/Biddeford office.

_____

Figure 6–6. Sample Completed Discharge Summary Indicating Types of Information to be Provided in each Space

CHAPTER 7

Marketing Your Work Hardening Program

Marketing is a phase of business about which medical professionals feel most uncomfortable. Because we are professionals providing a much needed service, we may feel that we shouldn't have to sell what we have to offer. However, potential customers, users of our services, usually do not know what we do. Therefore, we must educate them as to who we are, what we do, and how our service can help them.

SELLING YOUR PRODUCT

The first step in marketing is determining and defining your product. Then, define the product of your product! Your product is the offered service—in this case, work hardening. The product of your product is the result of the service provided—in this case, the return to work of injured workers. Do not be surprised if most of your customers are more interested in the results then in how you got there. One of the best methods for expanding your customer base through marketing is to offer services not expected or unique to your area. Go above and beyond the expected. Not only do you offer work hardening, but you also offer free parking, easy access, evening hours, and statistically proven results. You adjunct the work hardening program with job analysis performed by your staff, you teach back schools and upper-extremity cumulative trauma prevention classes both at your facility and to the industrial community. These are the expanded services that make your product more valuable to the consumer of your services. The current phrase for this is "value added." Basically, what you have done is offered a "generic product"— work hardening, which provides to consumers of your service the "expected product"—physical and psychosocial improvement. Then you started differentiating yourself from your competitors with your "expanded product"—the extras mentioned above. Market heavily those expanded products. You will never need to belittle a competitor if you use your assets. Besides, speaking ill of the competitor is very bad business. Instead speak positively about all of your strong points.

There is still one product not yet discussed—the "potential product." Here the sky is the limit! Few of us are fortunate enough to tap into this phase of our services. This includes products and services that adjunct your already expanded product. They could include progressive products and services never before seen or offered in your field. In the medical/industrial blend of services we generally have no tangible product to sell. We market our services.

With a service to offer, image sells your product. What kind of image do you want to conjure up when consumers hear about you? Most therapists say things like caring, knowledgeable, professional, energetic, and so forth. To this list you might add innovative, objective, hard working, and accommodating. No one else can decide for you the image you want to project. Marketing will be more difficult for you if you do not know how you want your company to be perceived. The words complete and thorough always come to my mind because I am such a stickler for attention to detail. Before deciding your marketing tactics, you should take some time to sit down and make a list of desirable images you want to portray. Separate the corporation's image from the individual professional's image. To market well, each professional's image of himself should blend with the desired corporate image.

How are you perceived and how do you want to be perceived? Probably not very many of us have stopped to ask this question, but it is important in marketing. Latest studies indicate that our image is projected 80% visually, 15% vocally, and only 5% by what we actually say! This means to get your foot in the door, you must first project the image visually. If this works, then you might actually get the opportunity to say something intelligent. Visual image can incorporate more than professional dress. It can include presentation of written material. Is it on letterhead? How does the logo look—is it dated? Are there spelling errors and typos? Is the sentence construction poor? Is the information presented incomplete? Visual image also can include facility presentation. Is it clean and modern? Is it organized? Is it set up to respect client's privacy? Is it safe? Does it reflect the philosophy of the program? If you preach functional orientation, do not fill the facility with high-tech equipment. Visual image also can include body language. Beware of closed body language (arms folded and legs crossed) if you want to project agreement and openness.

Voice projection should be clear and loud enough to be heard comfortably. Weak voices and upward inflections at the end of sentences reflect uncertainty in oneself and in what is being stated. State what you have to say with conviction. Use "I" statements whenever there is the chance that what you have to say will be taken negatively. For example, instead of saying "you made me feel unimportant when you did that to me" say "I felt unimportant when that happened." Assertive communications always win over aggressive ones. Acknowledging that an introductory handshake is one form of communication, use an assertive, firm grip. Wet fish handshakes and vise-grip handshakes say something negative about you. You want the handshake to be a customer's first positive impression of you.

Who Are Our Customers?

To decide how to sell to our customers we need to first determine who they are. Consider the following:

1. Patients/clients
2. Physicians
3. Insurance carriers
4. Vocational/rehabilitation counselors
5. Employers
6. Attorneys
7. Other health care providers
8. Workers' Compensation commissioners

These different disciplines require different approaches. We must speak their language. If their concern is cost savings, talk cost savings. The different agendas may include safety, efficacy, approach, results, timeliness of care, reliability of testing, and staffing ratios. Whatever the consumer's agenda, address it by asking yourself "what does my customer want and value?" Each customer wants to know that his individual needs will be met. Speaking with industry is much different than speaking with a medical colleague. If we expect other disciplines to listen to what we have to say, then we have a responsibility to learn from them what they need to know. In other words, what is the bottom line?

Size up your chances for success by surveying your strengths and weaknesses. Make a comparison worksheet. Consider the following:

1. Size of community and number of competitors
2. Referral base
3. Location convenience and visibility
4. Service hours
5. Specialty services offered
6. Cost/value
7. Staffing ratio/waiting list

Now highlight your strengths and decide if you can or want to compete with your competitor's strengths. Define your goals and determine what you want to offer, to whom you want to offer it, and how you will accomplish it. Write a mission statement. Your company mission will not become a reality until it is written down and shared. Mission statements are all-encompassing and oftentimes are very, very long sentences. Our company's mission statement says:

> MPTC's mission is to provide the highest quality service to the patients and clients in the community we serve and to our local, national, and international customers at a fair price in our acute care clinic and occupational injury prevention and rehabilitation programs through professional evaluation, treatment, and education, and a product line of slides, books, and seminars in order to promote a healthy society.

It is a mouthful! But what it makes clear is what we want to offer, to whom, and how. We even added who will benefit. It you have the opportunity to read other mission statements you will find that they are similar. The idea is to make your goals a reality by getting them written down. Then they will become clearer to you and your staff.

Marketing Events

Find any excuse you can to put your name in the public eye. It has become commonly accepted that people have to hear something five times before they remember it. So get your practice name into the public eye by using the following marketing events:

1. New employee
2. Practice expansion
3. New service
4. Course participation
5. Election to any professional or personal office
6. Awards, honors, and promotions

Marketing Formats

The longer you are in business, the more comfortable you become with certain marketing formats. The following is a list of suggested formats:

1. Letters, surveys, and reports
2. Folders, brochures, and informational flyers
3. Display board for use at trade shows and health fairs
4. Telephone calls
5. General press releases
6. Radio announcements
7. Newspaper display advertising
8. Company newsletter
9. Open house
10. Telephone directory
11. Fund-raising events in your community
12. Personal presentations
13. Imprinted courtesy items

You already may have used some of these formats so you know what works for you. If not, pick some that are appealing to you and go for it! If you already have found some you like, put a new twist on them and reuse them. For example, if you have found personal presentations work well for you, send out invitations on brown paper lunch bags to the medical community inviting them to a paper bag lunch series at your facility. Provide beverages and dessert and an informational hour on topics that you know will interest them. Share your expertise while publicizing your practice.

How Much Money Do I Need to Spend?

To determine how much money you will need to spend, first decide how much business you are trying to generate. Are you the new kid on the block or do you already have a reputation in the community through other work? If you are brand new and need to generate vast amounts of business, then you will need to be more elaborate and spend more. If you are unsure of the format that will give you the most "bang for your buck" in your area, tap resources such as the Service Core of Retired Executives (SCORE). These retired executives have a wealth of knowledge to share with small businesses just getting started or businesses that are expanding into uncharted waters.

To further determine the financial outlay, make a list of the people you are trying to reach with your marketing efforts. Then determine what advertising medium they would respond to. Do they like flash or are they more conservative? Tap your in-house resources. There are usually some very talented creative individuals within our own organizations who would be pleased to share their talents to help the marketing effort.

Remember that marketing is an ongoing process of fine-tuning your product and of keeping your customers informed. Everyone involved in the organization is involved in marketing, even informally. When employees share where they work an attitude is projected to the listener and marketing, good or bad, has taken place. In conclusion, the following suggestions may be helpful:

1. Keep your marketing style consistent with the image you want to project (high-tech, functional, etc.).
2. Each feature you highlight must have a relevant benefit to the customer. It must pass the "so what" test.
3. Do not market for more business than you can handle. It will ruin your reputation if the quality of your service suffers.
4. Do not degrade your competitors. Instead, highlight your strengths.
5. Avoid overuse of technical jargon. If they do not understand what you are talking about, the customers will lose interest.
6. Update your marketing materials as your image evolves.
7. Personal presentations should be free from offensive language.
8. Do not compromise your ethics and beliefs to gain a customer.
9. Gain ideas from what other successful companies have done.

The most important point to remember about marketing is that it is an ongoing process that needs constant attention. With that in mind, we might as well relax and enjoy the challenge.

STATISTICS

Beware of making the mistake that I made when I started the work hardening program. I decided that because I did not like to do statistics, I would just not worry about them. Wrong! The fact is that almost everyone involved with using your work hardening program will want to know how successful it has proven. How can you provide that kind of information when just starting out? Find out the success rate of the program or programs upon which you have built your work hardening program's philosophy. It is safe to assume that your program should be at least that successful. When asked about your success, make this statement of fact: "My program is patterned after the program at _____. Their studies indicate a success rate of _____%. Although our program is new, I believe that it will prove to be just as successful." You should say this in your own words, but have an answer prepared. You will be asked.

When speaking of statistics, almost anyone will tell you that you can make statistics say whatever you want. Bearing this in mind, when asking or reading about work hardening statistical success rates, investigate thoroughly exactly what those statistics are based on. Some facilities boast high return-to-work success rates when in fact the only clients they include in their studies are those who have entered the work hardening program, stayed for the complete course of treatment, and graduated. These facilities do not include any clients who began the program and dropped out. Because these clients are not included, it is like this segment of the population never existed. Statistics kept in this manner are the perfect example of making the statistics say whatever you want them to say. This statistical study reflects an inflated success rate unless it states exactly who is included in the results.

Statistics can be uncomplicated if you choose them to be. If you do not have access to a computer, a simple single form can suffice (Figure 7–1). It can be kept by hand. The important thing is to keep statistics from the very onset of your program. This form also can be filed as a tickler to follow-up with a telephone call in six months (or whatever time period you want to use) to determine the client's work status. At MPTC, we follow-up in six months to determine if the client is still in the workforce. A success at our facility is a client who returns to work and is still working six months later. All statistics are kept both manually and by computer. If you do not have access to a data base, check with your local university to see if there may be a graduate student interested in using your statistics to do a thesis. This will provide your facility with an excellent start and will provide the student with a unique opportunity.

Work-hardening success determination is critical to marketing, to improving on one's program, to the credibility of work hardening as an effective treatment mode, and to contributing to the research community the viability of work hardening. Work hardening makes sense on a gut level but the statistics must be available to prove it.

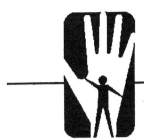
ERGONOMICS PLUS™
A Helping Hand with Injury Prevention and Rehabilitation

Name: _____   _____

Phone: (____) ____ – _____   Sex: M____   F_____

Date of Birth: ___/___/___   Date of Injury: ___/___/___

    Status: ____ Working
                    ____ Not Working Since: ___/___/___
                    ____ Not Looking
                    ____ Retired
                    ____ Other

Employer: _____

Occupation: _____

Injury Type: _____

Dominant: ____ Yes
                ____ No
                ____ N/A

Referral Source: _____

Figure 7–1.   Page 1 of 2

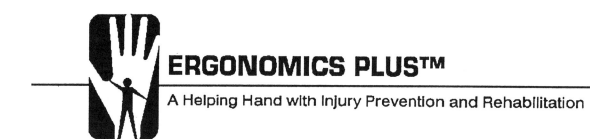

Physician: _____

Insurance Carrier: _____

Attorney: _____

Rehab. Counselor: _____

Assessment: _____

Date of Assessment: ___/___/___

Recommendation: _____

Program: _____

Date Entered: ___/___/___   Discharge Date: ___/___/___

Last Contact: ___/___/___   Present Status: ___ Working
                                                       ___ Not Working

Page 2 of 2

Figure 7–1.   (continued)

BIBLIOGRAPHIES

Compiled by Phyllis Quinn, M.Ed.
American Physical Therapy Association

A. Industrial Physical Therapy

A special news report on people and their jobs in offices, fields, and factories—Physical therapists help corporations pare health care costs. (Labor Letter) *Wall Street Journal*: 6 August 1985, 1.

Aiman P: Industry writing prescriptions for medical costs. *Iron Age* 1983; 226:26–43.

Baker KE: Health promotion. Promoting health to prevent disease. *Clin Manage in Phys Ther* 1984; 4(1):10–12.

Delacerda FG: A comparative study of three methods of treatment for shoulder girdle myofascial syndrome . . . work-induced. *J Orthop Sports Phys Ther* 1982; 4(1):51–54.

Driver R, Rafliff R: Employers' perceptions of benefits accrued from physical fitness programs. *Personnel Administrator* 1983; 37:1–67.

Fremion-Battell B: On the right track . . . Wellness programs can bail out hospitals. *Clin Manage in Phys Ther* 1985; 5(4):22–25.

Gottlieb A, Vandergoot D, Lutsky L: The role of the rehabilitation professional in corporate disability management. *J Rehabil* 1991; 57(2):23–28.

Hayne CR: The preventive role of physiotherapy in the national health service and industry. *Physiotherapy* 1988; 74(1):2–3.

Hebert LA: A change of place: opportunities in industry for physical therapists. *Clin Manage in Phys Ther* 1988; 8(6):5–8.

Hebert LA: Cumulative Trauma Prevention. *Clin Management* 1990; 10(5):30–34.

Hicks LL: Increasing role of economic analysis in the health care industry . . . cost effectiveness of providing physical therapy services. *Phys Ther* 1986; 66(10):1563–1566.

Huhn RR, Volski RV: Primary prevention programs for business and industry: role of physical therapists . . . promoting health and welfare. *Phys Ther* 1985; 65(12):1840–1844.

Jacobs B: Sound minds—sound bodies and savings. *Industry Week* 1983; 21:4067.

Johnston B, Blakney MG: Industrial health program: Alternative or obligation? *Clin Manage in Phys Ther* 1982; 2(4):18–20.

Kleven K: Taking health into our own hands: Preventive programs in industry. *Clin Manage in Phys Ther* 1982; 2(2):18–20.

Krug P, Wilson CR: Effectiveness of a pulmonary education program in reducing sick time in an employed population. (abstract) *Phys Ther* 1985; 65(5):712.

Lepore BA, Olson CN, Tommer GM: The dollars and sense of occupational back injury prevention training. *Clin Manage in Phys Ther* 1984; 4(2):38–42.

May VR, Stuart R, Soderberg G: Rehabilitating the injured worker: A physical capacity evaluation and work hardening model. (abstract) *Phys Ther* 1985; 65(5):738.

McManus K: Forced wellness? *Forbes* 1983; 132:11–246.

Molumphey MA, Unger B, Jensen GM, et al: Incidence of work-related low back pain in physical therapists. *Phys Ther* 1985; 65(4):482–486.

Morgan D: The industrial back patient: a physical therapist's perspective. *Topics in Acute Care and Trauma Rehabilitation* 1988; 2(4):38–46.

Olsheski J, Growick B: Industrial rehabilitation in the public sector: the Ohio experience. *J Rehabil* 1988; 54(2):46–49.

Rose SJ, Apts D, Strube M, et al: Identification of work tasks related to back pain in coal miners. (abstract) *Phys Ther* 1985; 65(5):672.

Thomas LK, Hislop HJ, Waters RL: Physiological work performance in chronic low back disability: Effects of a progressive activity program. *Phys Ther* 1980; 60:407–411.

Twelves JW: Physical Therapy in Industry. *Clin Management* 1990; 10(5):14–16, 19.

Volski R: How to convince management to start a corporate fitness program. *Clin Manage in Phys Ther* 1982; 2(4):13–17.

Volski R: Organization of a physical fitness program for business or industry. *Clin Manage in Phys Ther* 1982; 2(2):21–27.

B. Work Hardening

Anderson L: Educational approaches to management of low back pain. *Orthoped Nurs* 1989; 8(1):43–46.

Benner CL, Schilling AD, Klein L: Coordinated teamwork in California industrial rehabilitation. *J Hand Surg* 1987; 12(5 Pt 2):936–939.

Caruso LA, Chan DE, Chan A: The management of work-related back pain. *Am J Occup Ther* 1987; 41(2):112–117.

Cooper J, Quanbury A, Grahame R, Dubo H: Trunk kinematics and trunk muscle EMG activity during five functional locomotor types. *Canadian J Occup Ther* 1989; 56(3):120–127.

Haig AJ, Penha S: Worker rehabilitation programs. Separating face from fiction. *Western J Med* 1991; 154(5):528–531.

Holmes D: The role of the occupational therapist-work evaluator. *Am J Occup Ther* 1985; 39(5):308–313.

Johnston B, Blakney MG: Industrial health program: Alternative or obligation? *Clin Manage in Phys Ther* 1982; 2(4):18–20.

Kleven K: Taking health into our own hands: Preventive programs in industry. *Clin Manage in Phys Ther* 1982; 2(2):18–20.

Leman CJ: An approach to work hardening in burn rehabilitation. *Topics in Acute Care and Trauma Rehab* 1987; 1(4):62–73.

Lepping V: Work hardening: a valuable resource for the occupational health nurse. *AAOHN J* 1990; 38(7):313–317.

Lepore BA, Olson CN, Tommer GM: The dollars and sense of occupational back injury prevention training. *Clin Manage in Phys Ther* 1984; 4(2):38–42.

Matheson LN, Ogden LD, Violette K, et al: Work hardening: Occupational therapy in industrial rehabilitation. *Am J Occup Ther* 1985; 39(5):314–321.

May VR, Stuart R, Soderburg G: Rehabilitating the injured worker: A physical capacity evaluation and work hardening model. (abstract) *Phys Ther* 1985; 65(5):738.

McElligott J, Miscovich SJ, Fielding LP: Low back injury in industry: the value of a recovery program. *Connecticut Med* 1989; 53(12):711–715.

Pedersen DM, Clark JA, Johns RE, Jr, et al: Quantitative muscle strength testing: A comparison of job strength requirements and actual worker strength among military technicians. *Milit Med* 1989; 154(1):14–18.

Peters P: Successful return to work following a musculoskeletal injury. *AAOHN J* 1990; 38(6):264–270.

Puffer JC, et al: Management of overuse injuries. *Am Fam Phys* 1988; 38(3):225–232.

Ryden LA, Molgaard CA, Bobbitt SL: Benefits of a back care and light duty health promotion program in a hospital setting. *J Commun Health* 1988; 13(4):222–230.

Swarts AD, et al: Tissue pressure management in the vocational setting. *Arch Phys Med Rehabil* 1988; 69(2):97–100.

Taylow ME: Return to work following back surgery: a review. *Am J Industrial Med* 1989; 16(1):79–88.

Thomas LK, Hislop HJ, Waters RL: Physiological work performance in chronic low back disability. Effects of a progressive activity program. *Phys Ther* 1980; 60:407–411.

Tollison CD, Satterthwaite JR, Kriegel ML, et al: Interdisciplinary treatment of low back pain. A clinical outcome comparison of compensated versus non-compensated groups. *Orthoped Rev* 1990; 19(8): 701–706.

Tramposh AK: Work-related therapy for the injured reduces return-to-work barriers. *Occup Health Safety* 1988; 57(4):55–56, 82.

Wilson S, Mejia D: Work hardening: Back disabilities take on a new dimension. *Topics in Acute Care and Trauma Rehab* 1980; 2(4):73–83.

Work hardening: Bridging the gap. *Optimal Health* 1988; 4(3):42–44.

Work hardening guidelines . . . in an occupational therapy setting. *Am J Occup Ther* 1986; 40(12):841–843.

Work hardening guidelines (position paper). *Am J Occup Ther* 1986; 40(12):841–843.

Wyrick JM, Niemeyer LD, Ellexson M, et al: Occupational therapy work-hardening programs: a demographic study. *Am J Occup Ther* 1991; 45(2):109–112.

C. Marketing

Boynton PS, Fiar PA: Becoming a market-driven rehabilitation program: A case study. *Rehabil Lit* 1986; 47(7–8):174–178.

Brown GD: Changing health environments—implications for physical therapy research, education, and practice: A special communication. *Phys Ther* 1986; 66(8):1242–1245.

Carey RG, Seibert JH: Integrating program evaluation, quality assurance, and marketing for inpatient rehabilitation . . . the LORS American Data System (LADS). *Rehabil Nurs* 1988; 13(2):66–70.

Crocker KE, Alden J: An investigation of clients' and practitioners' views of the effect of physical therapy advertising and its content. *J Health Care Mark* 1986; 6(3):12–18.

Fremion-Batelli B: On the right track . . . Wellness programs can bail out hospitals. *Clin Manage Phys Ther* 1985; 5(4):22–25.

Gottlieb A, Vandergoot D, Lutsky L: The role of the rehabilitation professional in corporate disability mangement. *J Rehabil* 1991; 57(2):23–28.

Grubbs N, Reese NB: Marketing physical therapy. *Clin Management* 1991; 11(5):40–44.

Horting M: Insurance reimbursement and the physical therapist. Marketing strategies: How to enhance reimbursement for PT services. *Clin Manage Phys Ther* 1987; 7(2):36–37.

House SG: Advertising and the individual professional. *Clin Manage Phys Ther* 1982; 2(3):33–35.

Marketing your pulmonary rehabilitation program. *AARTIMES* 1983; 7(1):44–45.

Nadolsky JM: The marketing of rehabilitation services. *J Rehabil* 1984; 50(3):4–5. 66–67.

Novak S: Entering the marketing area. *Rehabil Nurs* 1987; 12(4):176.

Panos A: Professional advertising . . . physical therapists. *Clin Manage Phys Ther* 1982; 2(3):36–37.

Powells S: Marketing rehab: Not just another ad effort. *Hospitals* 1987; 61(18):38–39.

Sabin S: Rehab program's marketing plan was tailored to fit. *Nurs Health Care* 1985; 6(5):268–271.

Schaefer K: An objective eye . . . finding your clinic's marketing niche requires a periodic assessment. *Clin Manage Phys Ther* 1988; 8(5):6–9.

Special marketing wrap-up. *Hospitals* 1984; 58(12):33–34, 38–46, 56–62.

Stevens A: Public relations: A powerful marketing tool for the PT. *Clin Manage Phys Ther* 1985; 5(5):24–25.

Tanner SE, Klein JB: Market analysis reveals rehab program potential. *Hospitals* 1985; 59(11):65–66.

Daily Schedules

Date	4-6	4-7	4-8	4-9	4-10	4-13	4-14	4-15	4-16
Hours	2 hrs.	2 hrs.	2 hrs.	2 hrs.	2 hrs.	4 hrs.	2 hrs.	4 hrs.	2 hrs.
Upper Body Warm-Up ★	orien-tation	10x	10x	10x	10x	10x	10x	10x	10x
Lower Body Warm-Up	orien-tation	10x	10x	10x	10x	10x	10x	10x	10x
Back Exercises	screening	stress mgmt.	10x	10x	stress mgmt.	10x	stress mgmt.	10x	15x •
Treadmill	screening	stress mgmt.	Dyno hr.	5 min.	stress mgmt.	7 min. •	stress mgmt.	Dyno hr.	7 min.
Lower Extremity Exercises	screening		Dyno hr.	10x	back ex. 10x	10x (break)	back ex. 10x	(break)	10x
Circuit I						45 min.		45 min.	
Upper Extremity Exercises						10x		10x	
Ergonomic Bike						5 min.		5 min.	
Cool Downs ✓						5x		5x	

Name_____ Ben D. Nees _____

Daily Schedule 1: Back Injured Client

Sample Daily Schedule for Back Patient showing Dates at the top of the page and number of hours client is spending for Work Hardening for those days

Date	4/17	4/20	4/21	4/22	4/23	4/24		4/27	
Hours	4 hrs.	4 hrs.	4 hrs.	4 hrs.	4 hrs.	6 hrs.		6 hrs.	
Upper Body Warm-Up ★	10x	10x	10x	10x	10x	10x	Circuit 30 min.	10x	Circuit 30 min. I
Lower Body Warm-Up	10x	10x	10x	10x	10x	10x	row 5 min.●	10x	row 5 min.
Back Exercises	stress mgmt.	15x	stress mgmt.	15x	15x	stress mgmt.	cool downs (5x)	15x	cool downs 5x
Treadmill	stress mgmt.	10 min.	stress mgmt.	Dyno hour	12 min.●	stress mgmt.		12 min.	8 min.
Circuit I	30 min. (break)	30 min. (break)	30 min. (break)	Dyno hour (break)	30 min. (break)	30 min. (break)		30 min. (break)	10x
Lower Extremity Exercises	15x ●	15x	15x	15x	15x	15x		15x	
Upper Extremity Exercises	10x	10x	10x	10x	10x	10x		10x	
Ergonomic Bike	7 min.	7 min.	10 min.●	10 min.	10 min.	10 min.		10 min.	
Circuit II	45 min.	45 min.	45 min.	45 min.	45 min.	60 min.● (break)		60 min. (break)	
Cool Downs ✓	5x	5x	5x	5x	5x	counter 30 min.		counter 30 min.	
Walk and Carry						walk and carry 10# 15 min.		walk and carry 10# 15 min.	

Daily Schedule 1: Back Injured Client (continued)

Sample Daily Schedule for Back Patient showing Dates at the top of the page and number of hours client is spending for Work Hardening for those days

Name_____ Ben D. Nees _____

Date	4/28		4/29		4/30		5/1		
Hours	6 hrs.		6 hrs.		6 hrs.		6 hrs.		
Upper Body Warm-Up ★	10x	circuit 30 min. I	10x	circuit 30 min. I	10x	circuit 30 min. I	10x	circuit 30 min. I	
Lower Body Warm-Up	10x	cool down 5x	10x	row 5 min.•	10x	row 5 min.	10x	row 5 min. (break)	
Back Exercises	stress mgmt.		20x•	cool down 5x	20x	cool down 5x	stress mgmt.	counter 60 min. II	
Treadmill	stress mgmt.		Dyno hr.		12 min.		stress mgmt.	cool down 5x	
Circuit I	30 min. (break)		Dyno hr. (break)		30 min. I (break)		30 min. (break)		
Lower Extremity Exercises	15x		15x		15x		15x		
Upper Extremity Exercises	10x		10x		10x		10x		
Ergonomic Bike	10 min.		10 min.		10 min.		10 min.		
Circuit II	60 min. (lunch)		60 min. (lunch)		60 min. (lunch)		60 min. (lunch)		
Counter	1/2 hr.		1/2 hr.		1/2 hr.		1/2 hr.		
Walk and Carry Stair Climbing	10# 15 min.		10# 15 min.		10# 15 min.		10# each hand 15 min.		

Daily Schedule 1: Back Injured Client (continued)

Sample Daily Schedule for Back Patient showing Dates at the top of the page and number of hours client is spending for Work Hardening for those days

Name_____ Ben D. Nees _____

Date	5/4		5/5		5/6		5/7		
Hours	8 hrs.		8 hrs.		8 hrs.		8 hrs.		
Upper Body Warm-Up *	10x	circuit 30 min. I	10x	circuit 30 min. I	10x	circuit 30 min. I	10x	circuit 30 min. I	
Lower Body Warm-Up	10x	row 5 min. (break)	10x	row 5 min. (break)	10x	row 5 min. (break)	10x	row 5 min. (break)	
Back Exercises	20x	counter 30 min.	stress mgmt.	counter 30 min.	20x	counter 30 min.	20x	counter 30 min.	
Treadmill	15 min.•	circuit 60 min. II	stress mgmt.	circuit 60 min. II	Dyno hr.	circuit 60 min. II	15 min.	circuit 60 min. II	
Circuit I	30 min. (break)	cool down 5x	30 min.	cool down 5x	Dyno hr.	cool down 5x	30 min. circuit (break)	cool down 5x	
Lower Extremity Exercises	15x		15x		15x		15x		
Upper Extremity Exercises	10x		10x		10x		10x		
Ergonomic Bike	12 min.•		12 min.		12 min.		12 min.		
Circuit II	60 min. (lunch)		60 min. (lunch)		60 min. (lunch)		60 min. (lunch)		
Counter	1/2 hr.		1/2 hr.		1/2 hr.		1/2 hr.		
Walk and Carry Stair Climbing	10# each hand 15 min.		10# each hand 15 min.		10# each hand 15 min.		10# each hand 15 min.		

Daily Schedule 1: Back Injured Client (continued)

Name_____ Ben D. Nees _____

Sample Daily Schedule for Back Patient showing Dates at the top of the page and number of hours client is spending for Work Hardening for those days

Date	8/1	8/2	8/3	8/4	8/5	8/8	8/9	8/10	8/11
Hours	2 hrs.	2 hrs.	2 hrs.	2 hrs.	2 hrs.	2 hrs.	2 hrs.	2 hrs.	2 hrs.
Upper Body Warm-Up *	NMSS	10x	10x	10x	10x	10x	10x	10x	10x
Theraband	NMSS	10x	10x	10x	10x	10x	10x	10x	10x
Lower Body Exercises	orien-tation	stress mgmt. 45 min.	10x	10x	stress mgmt. 45 min.	10x	stress mgmt. 45 min.	10x	10x
Ergonomic Bike (Push/Pull only)	orien-tation	5 min.	5 min.	7 min.•	stress mgmt. 45 min.	7 min.	7 min.	8 min.•	8 min.
Upper Extremity Exercises	orien-tation	cage levels 5-6-7	Dyno hr.	10x	cage levels 5-6-7	10x wts. added, see ex's •	cage levels 5-6-7	10x	10x
		no cage done due to heat		CA					

Daily Schedule 2: Extremity Injured Client

Sample Daily Schedule for Upper Extremity Injured Client

Name_____Carrie Proppa_____

Date	8/12	8/13	8/16	8/17	8/18	8/19	8/22	8/23	8/24
Hours	4 hrs.	4 hrs.	4 hrs.	4 hrs.	4 hrs.	6 hrs.	6 hrs.	4 hrs.	6 hrs.
Upper Body Warm-Up *	10x	10x	10x	10x	10x	10x	10x	10x	10x
Theraband	10x	10x	10x	10x	10x	10x	10x	10x	10x
Lower Body Exercises	stress mgmt.	10x	stress mgmt.	10x	10x	stress mgmt.	10x	stress mgmt.	10x
Bike	stress mgmt.	10 min.	stress mgmt.	Dyno hr.	10 min.	stress mgmt/	60 min. circuit I (break)	stress mgmt.	Dyno hr. (break)
Upper Extremity Exercises	circuit I 30 min. (break)	10x (break)	circuit I 30 min. (break)	Dyno hr. (break)	15x • (break)	circuit I 30 min. (break)	bike 10 min.	circuit I 30 min. (break)	bike 10 min.
Cage	5-6-7	5-6-7	5-6-7	5-6-7	5-6-7	UE Ex. 15x	UE Ex. 15x	5-6-7	UE Ex. 15x
Circuit	upper extrem. ex. 10x	45 min.	upper extrem. ex. 10x	60 min.	60 min.	upper extrem. ex. 15x	circuit II 60 min.	upper extrem. ex. 15x	circuit I 60 min.
Body Ball Exercises	10	10x	10x			lunch 30 min.	lunch 30 min.	10x body ball	lunch 30 min.
Lower Extremity Exercises	10x	10x	15x •	15x	15x	circuit II 60 min.	counter 30 min.	15x LE exercises	counter 30 min.
Cool Downs ✓	5x	5x	5x	5x	5x	cool down	circuit I 60 min. cool down	5x cool down	circuit I 60 min. cool down
							CA		

Daily Schedule 2: Extremity Injured Client (continued)

Name_____ Carrie Proppa _____

Sample Daily Schedule with Increasing
Hours for Upper Extremity Injured Client

Date	8/25	8/26	8/29	8/30	8/31	9/1		9/2	
Hours	6 hrs.	6 hrs.	6 hrs.	6 hrs.	6 hrs.	8 hrs.	cont.	8 hrs.	cont.
Upper Body Warm-Up ∗	10x	10x	10x	10x	10x	10x	(break) 15 min.	10x	(break) 15 min.
Theraband	10x	10x	10x	10x	10x	10x	body ball 10x	10x	body ball
Lower Body Exercises	10x	stress mgmt.	10x	stress mgmt.	10x	10x	counter 30 min.	stress mgmt.	counter 30 min.
Circuit	60 min. I (break)	lower body stretch (break)	60 min. I (break)	lower body stretch (break)	Dyno (break)	60 min. I (break)	lower extrem. ex. 15x	30 min. I	lower extrem. ex. 15x
Ergonomic Bike (Push/ Pull only)	10 min.	10 min.	10 min.	10 min.	10 min.	10 min.	circuit II 30 min.	10 min.	circuit 30 min.
Upper Extremity Exercises	15x	15x	15x	15x	15x	15x	cool downs 5x	15x	cool downs 5x
Circuit	60 min. II	60 min. I	60 min. II	60 min. I	60 min. I	60 min. II		60 min. II	only • stayed 4 hrs.
Lunch	30 min.	30 min.	30 min.	30 min.	30 min.	30 min.		30 min.	
Counter	30 min.	30 min.	30 min.	30 min.	30 min.	30 min.		30 min.	
Circuit	60 min. I 5x cool down	60 min. II 5x cool down	60 min. I 5x cool down	60 min. II 5x cool down	60 min. I 5x cool down	60 min. II		60 min. II	

Daily Schedule 2: Extremity Injured Client (continued)

Name_____ Carrie Proppa _____

Sample Daily Schedule with Increasing Hours for Upper Extremity Injured Client

Date	9/5		9/6		9/7		9/8		
Hours	8 hrs.	cont.	8 hrs.	cont.	8 hrs.	cont.	8 hrs.	cont.	
Upper Body Warm-Up ★	10x	(break) 15 min.	10x	(break) 15 min.	10x	(break) 15 min.	10x	(break) 15 min.	
Theraband	10x	walk 15 min. carry bilat.	10x	walk 15 min. carry bilat.	10x	walk 15 min. carry bilat.	10x	walk 15 min. carry bilat.	
Lower Body Exercises	10x	counter 30 min.	stress mgmt.	counter 30 min.	10x	counter 30 min.	10x	counter 30 min.	
Circuit	60 min. I (break)	lower extrem. ex. 15x	30 min. I (break)	lower extrem. ex. 15x	Dyno (break)	lower extrem. ex. 15x	60 min. I • (break)	lower extrem. ex. 15x	
Ergonomic Bike	10 min.	circuit 30 min. II	10 min.	circuit 30 min. II	10 min.	circuit 30 min. I	10 min.	circuit 30 min. II	
Upper Extremity Exercises	15x	cool downs 5x	15x	cool downs 5x	15x	cool downs 5x	15x	cool downs 5x	
Circuit	60 min. II		60 min. II		60 min. I				60 min. II	
Lunch	30 min.		30 min.		30 min.				30 min.	
Counter	30 min.		30 min.		30 min.				30 min.	
Circuit	60 min. I		60 min. I		60 min. II				60 min.	

Daily Schedule 2: Extremity Injured Client (continued)

Name _____ Carrie Proppa _____

Sample Daily Schedule Activities in Work Hardening Program with Increasing Hours for Upper Extremity Injured Client

Exercises

Appendix B contains examples of exercises utilized by MPTC in our work hardening program. The exercises are muscle specific and include warm-ups, upper extremity exercises, lower body exercises and cool downs. Many of these exercises are referred to in the Daily Schedules in Appendix A.

They are included here to provide a general time frame for the therapeutic exercise section of most work hardening clients. In an acute care therapy, a program such as this would be too time consuming. However, since the work hardening client spends from two to eight hours per day in the program, a comprehensive warm-up, strengthening and cool down is frequently necessary.

Each exercise is illustrated and accompanied by simple instructions. We have found that this ensures client involvement and cooperation and time savings for both client and therapist.

Asterisks and check marks found on some of the exercises correspond to those on the Daily Schedules.

Neck Flexion—Isometric ★
Clasp hands on forehead, try to touch chin to chest, resisting motion with hands. Do not hold breath.
Hold _____ counts.
Repeat _____ times.

Neck Axial Extension—Isometric ★
Clasp hands behind head. Try to look up at ceiling, resisting motion with hands. Do not hold breath.
Hold _____ counts.
Repeat _____ times.

Neck Rotation—Isometric ★
Place hand on right side of head. Try to turn head to right, resisting motion with hand. Do not hold breath.
Hold _____ counts.
Repeat _____ times.

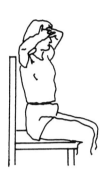
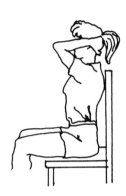
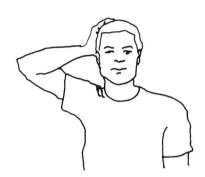

Neck—Active ★
Flexion—Curl chin to chest.
Axial extension—tuck chin in.
Do not tip head up or down.
Rotation—Tuck chin in. Turn head to look over right shoulder and then look over left shoulder.
Sidebending—Tilt head to right shoulder and then to left.
Hold _____ counts.
Repeat _____ times.

Neck Lateral Flexion—Isometric ★
Hand on right side of head. Try to move right ear to shoulder, resisting motion with hand. Do not hold breath.
Hold _____ counts.
Repeat to left side and hold.
Repeat _____ times.

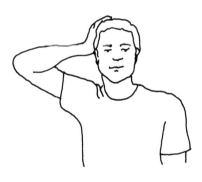

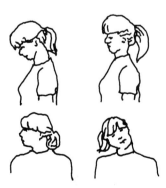

**Trunk extension—Prone on ★
Elbows**
Lie on stomach, prop up on elbows.
Hold _____ counts/minutes.
Repeat _____ times.

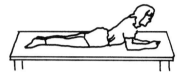

Trunk Extension—Press-Up
Lie on stomach, hands beside
shoulders. Straighten arms, raising
chest up. Keep waistline on mat.
Repeat _____ times.

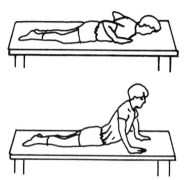

Trunk Extension—Active
Lying on stomach, raise left arm and
right leg.
Hold _____ counts.
Raise right arm and left leg and hold.
Repeat _____ times.

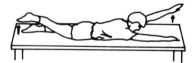

Trunk Extension—Positioned ★
Lie on stomach, place pillow(s) under
chest. Remain in position for _____
minutes.
Repeat _____ times per day.

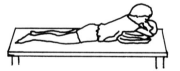

Trunk Extension—Active
Begin on hands and knees. Lift right arm and leg. Do not arch back.
Hold ____ counts.
Lift left arm and leg and hold.
Repeat ____ times.

Trunk Extension—Backbends ✱
Stand with hands on hips. Lean backward. Keep knees straight.
Hold ____ counts.
Repeat ____ times.

Trunk Extension—Stretching ✱
Begin on hands and knees. Sit back on heels, keeping hand placement. Stretch is felt in back.
Hold ____ counts.
Repeat ____ times.

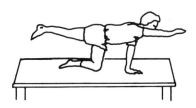
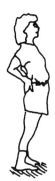
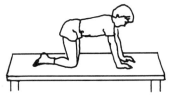
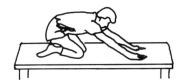

Trunk Flexion—Posterior Pelvic Tilt
Lie on back, knees bent and feet flat. Tighten stomach, tilting hips and flattening lower back.
Hold ____ counts.
Repeat ____ times.

Trunk Flexion—Single Knee to Chest
Lie on back, knees bent with feet flat. Raise left knee to chest, holding back of thigh with hand.
Hold ____ counts.
Repeat with right leg and hold.
Repeat ____ times.
Progress to beginning with legs straight.

Trunk Flexion—Double Knee to Chest
Lie on back, knees bent and feet flat. Raise knees to chest, holding back of thighs with hands.
Hold ____ counts.
Repeat ____ times.

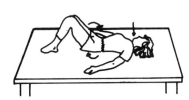
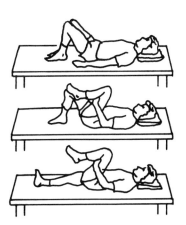
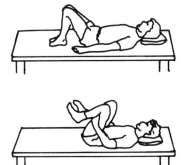

Trunk Flexion—Cat and Camel
Begin on hands and knees. Sag back
and raise head.
Hold _____ counts.
Lower head and arch back and hold.
Repeat _____ times.

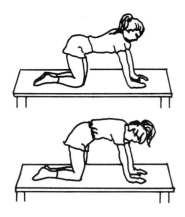

Trunk Rotation—Active
Lie on back, knees bent and feet flat.
Lower knees to left.
Hold _____ counts.
Lower knees to right and hold.
Repeat _____ times.

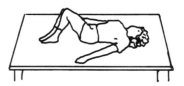

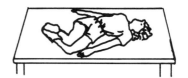

Trunk Rotation—Diagonal Partial
Sit-up
Lie on back, knees bent and feet flat.
Curl head and chest, reaching hands
to right side. Raise shoulder blades
only.
Hold _____ counts.
Reach to left side and hold.
Repeat _____ times.

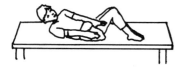

Trunk Lateral Flexion—Stretching ✓
Hands on hips. Reach right arm over
head. Stretch is felt on side.
Hold _____ counts.
Repeat to left side and hold.
Repeat _____ times.

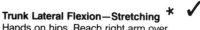

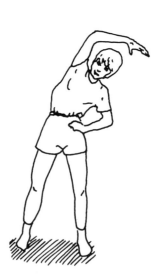

Scapular Elevation—Shoulder ✳ ✔
Circles
Roll shoulders backward.
Repeat _____ times.
Roll shoulders forward.
Repeat _____ times.

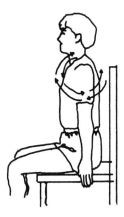

Scapular Elevation—Active ✳
Shrug shoulders.
Hold _____ counts.
Repeat _____ times.
Progress to _____ lbs. at wrists/hands.

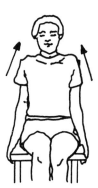

Scapular Adduction—Active ✳
Pinch shoulder blades together.
Do not shrug shoulders.
Hold _____ counts.
Repeat _____ times.

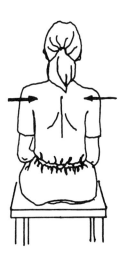

Shoulder Flexion—Active
Lie on back, lift _____ arm over
head with thumb up and elbow
straight.
Hold _____ counts.
Repeat _____ times.
Progress to _____ lbs. at wrist/hand.

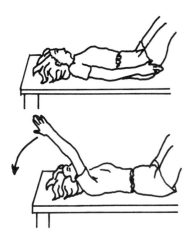

Shoulder Flexion—Active
Lift _____ arm over head with
thumb up and elbow straight.
Hold _____ counts.
Repeat _____ times.
Progress to _____ lbs. at wrist/hand.

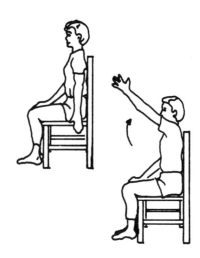

Shoulder Flexion—Resistive
Hold tubing in hands. Raise _____
hand over head with thumb up.
Hold _____ counts.
Repeat _____ times.

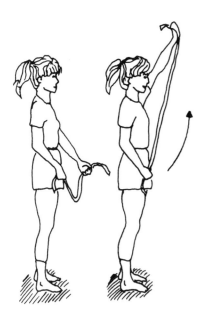

Shoulder Flexion—Resistive
Standing, tubing under foot, holding
other end with _____ hand. Raise
arm with thumb up and elbow straight.
Hold _____ counts.
Repeat _____ times.

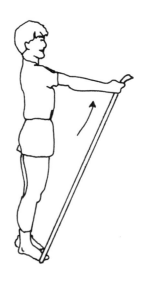

Shoulder Medial Rotation— ✔
Self-Range of Motion
Hands over lower back. Slide hands
up to shoulder blades. Do not lean
forward.
Hold ____ counts.
Repeat ____ times.

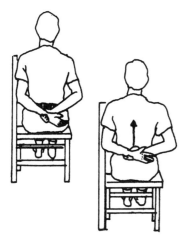

**Shoulder Medial and Lateral
Rotation—Active**
Lie on ____ side with forearm on
stomach. Lift ____ hand up.
Keep elbow bent at side.
Hold ____ counts.
Repeat ____ times.
Progress to ____ lbs. at wrist/hand.

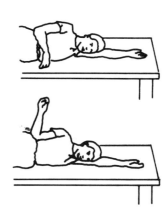

**Shoulder Medial and Lateral
Rotation—Active**
Lie on stomach, ____ arm out to
side with elbow bent and towel roll
under arm. Move hand backward with
palm up.
Hold ____ counts.
Move hand forward with palm down
and hold.
Repeat ____ times.
Progress to ____ lbs. at wrist/hand.

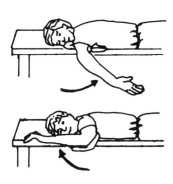

Shoulder Rotation—Inferior Cuff ✔ ★
Stretch
____ hand behind back and
opposite hand on elbow. Pull arm to
opposite side. Stretch is felt on side
and shoulder.
Hold ____ counts/minutes.
Repeat ____ times.

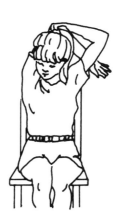

**Horizontal Shoulder Adduction—
Active**
Lie on stomach, _____ arm off
mat with elbow bent. Raise arm off
mat. Do not raise chest.
Hold _____ counts.
Repeat _____ times.
Progress to _____ lbs. at wrist/hand.

**Horizontal Shoulder Abduction and
Adduction—Active**
_____ arm out to side at shoulder
height. Reach hand to opposite
shoulder. Keep elbow straight.
Hold _____ counts.
Repeat _____ times.
Progress to _____ lbs. at wrist/hand.

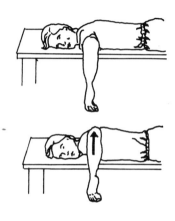

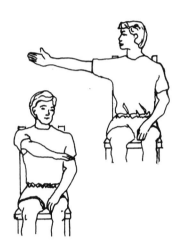

**Horizontal Shoulder Adduction— ✳
Stretching**
Stand in corner with forearms on wall.
Lean chest to wall. Stretch is felt in chest.
Hold _____ counts.
Repeat _____ times.

**Horizontal Shoulder Abduction—
Stretching**
_____ arm across chest with opposite
hand on elbow. Pull arm across chest.
Stretch is felt in back of arm and shoulder.
Hold _____ counts.
Repeat _____ times.

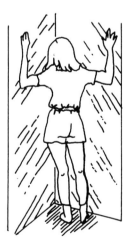

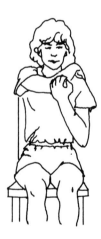

Shoulder Abduction—Arm Circles ✔
Arms out to side at shoulder height.
Move arms in a circle, clockwise.
Repeat _____ times.
Move arms counterclockwise.
Repeat _____ times.

Shoulder Abduction—Resistive
Hands at mid-thigh and thumbs
pointing down. Hold _____ lbs. in
hands. Raise arms, but not greater
than shoulder height.
Hold _____ counts.
Repeat _____ times.

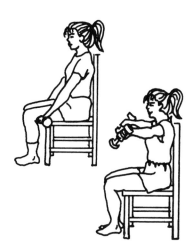

Shoulder Adduction—Stretching
Stand with _____ side to wall and
_____ arm on wall. Move body to
wall, reaching hand to ceiling.
Stretch is felt under shoulder.
Hold _____ counts.
Repeat _____ times.

Shoulder Extension—Active
Lie on stomach lift _____ arm up.
Keep elbow straight.
Hold _____ counts.
Repeat _____ times.
Progress to _____ lbs. at wrist/hand.

Shoulder Extension—Self-Range ★
of Motion
Clasp hands behind back. Move
hands away from bottom. Keep
elbows straight. Do not lean forward.
Hold _____ counts.
Repeat _____ times.

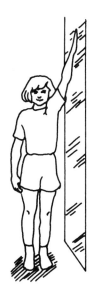

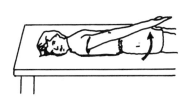

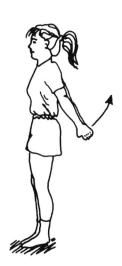

Shoulder Extension—Resistive
Tubing above elbows with arms at
shoulder height. Lower _____ arm
with elbow straight. Keep opposite
arm still.
Hold _____ counts.
Repeat _____ times.
Progress to placing tubing at forearms.

Shoulder Extension—Stretching
Stand with _____ arm on wall
above head. Move body to wall,
reaching hand to ceiling. Stretch is felt
under shoulder.
Hold _____ counts.
Repeat _____ times.

Shoulder Extension—Resistive
Hold tubing over head with thumbs
up. Lower _____ arm with elbow
straight. Keep opposite arm above
head.
Hold _____ counts.
Repeat _____ times.

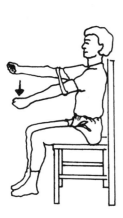
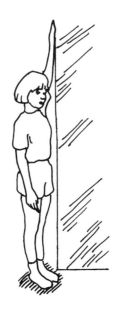
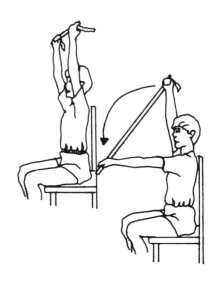

**Elbow Flexion and Extension—
Active**
Bend _____ elbow.
Hold _____ counts.
Straighten elbow and hold.
Repeat _____ times.
Progress to _____ lbs. at wrist/hand.

**Elbow Flexion and Extension—
Resistive**
Tubing on forearms, palms up. Bend
_____ elbow. Keep opposite
forearm still.
Hold _____ counts.
Straighten elbow and hold.
Repeat _____ times.

Elbow Flexion—Resistive
Sitting, tubing on chair leg. Hold
tubing in _____ hand. Bend elbow.
Hold _____ counts.
Repeat _____ times.

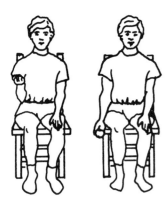
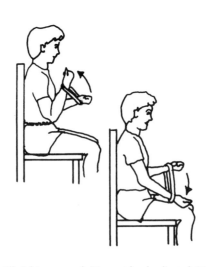
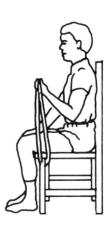

Elbow Extension—Active ✓
_____ arm above head, elbow pointing to ceiling. Straighten elbow.
Hold _____ counts.
Repeat _____ times.
Progress to _____ lbs. at wrist/hand.

Forearm Supination—Resistive
Hold tubing with palms down, elbows at sides. Turn palms up.
Hold _____ counts.
Repeat _____ times.

Forearm Pronation—Resistive
Hold tubing with palms up, elbows at sides. Turn palms down.
Hold _____ counts.
Repeat _____ times.

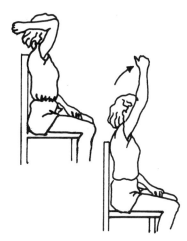
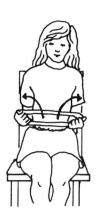
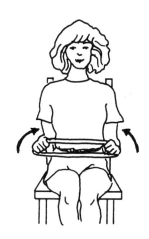

Wrist Flexion and Extension—Resistive
Sitting, _____ forearm on table, palm up. Tubing under foot and hold other end in hand. Raise hand up.
Hold _____ counts.
Turn palm down. Raise hand up and hold.
Repeat _____ times.

Hip Abduction—Active
Lie on _____ side with bottom knee bent. Raise top leg. Keep knee straight and toes pointed forward. Do not let top hip roll backward.
Hold _____ counts.
Repeat _____ times.
Progress to _____ lbs. at thigh/ankle.

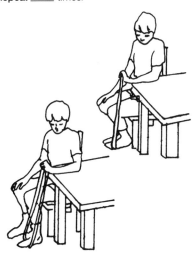
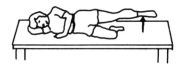

Hip Extension—Bridging
Lie on back, knees bent and feet flat.
Lift bottom up.
Hold _____ counts.
Repeat _____ times.

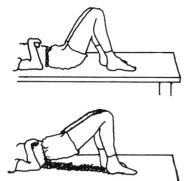

Hip Extension—Active
Lie on stomach, towel roll under
_____ thigh. Raise hip up with
knee bent. Do not raise hip.
Hold _____ counts.
Repeat _____ times.
Progress to _____ lbs. at thigh/ankle.

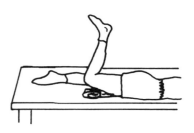

Hip Extension—Active
Begin on hands and knees. Straighten
_____ leg.
Hold _____ counts.
Repeat _____ times.
Progress to _____ lbs. at thigh/ankle.

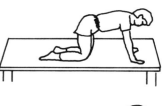
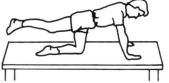

Hip Extension—Active
Begin on hands and knees. Lift
_____ leg with knee bent and heel
pointing to ceiling.
Hold _____ counts.
Repeat _____ times.
Progress to _____ lbs. at thigh/ankle.

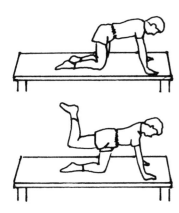

Hip Extension—Gluteal Set
Squeeze bottom together. Do not hold
breath.
Hold _____ counts.
Repeat _____ times.

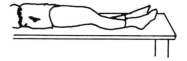

Hip Adduction—Active
Lie on _____ side, top leg on
chair. Raise bottom leg to chair seat.
Hold _____ counts.
Repeat _____ times.
Progress to _____ lbs. at thigh/ankle.

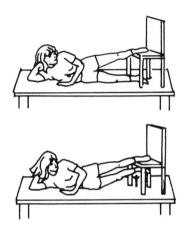

Hip Adduction—Active
Lie on _____ side. Place top leg
behind bottom leg. Raise bottom leg
up. Stay on side with toes pointed forward.
Hold _____ counts.
Repeat _____ times.
Progress to _____ lbs. at thigh/ankle.

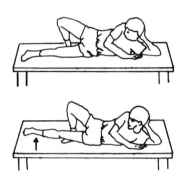

Hip Adduction—Stretching
Sit with feet together. Move heels to
groin. Stretch is felt on inside of thighs.
Hold _____ counts.
Repeat _____ times.

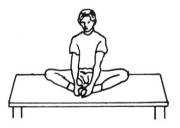

Hip Abduction—Stretching
Lie on back, move left knee across
right leg to mat. Keep shoulders flat
on mat. Stretch is felt on outside of thigh.
Hold _____ counts.
Repeat on opposite side and hold.
Repeat _____ times.

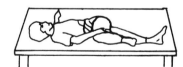

Hip Abduction—Stretching

Sitting, cross left leg over right. Place right elbow on outside of left knee. Turn body to left using elbow to push left knee in. Stretch is felt on outside of thigh.
Hold _____ counts.
Repeat to opposite side and hold.
Repeat _____ times.

Knee Extension—Straight Leg Raise

Lie on back, _____ knee bent and foot flat. Lift opposite leg up one foot. Keep knee straight and toes pointed up.
Hold _____ counts.
Repeat _____ times.
Progress to _____ lbs. at thigh/ankle.

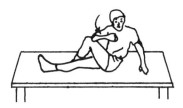

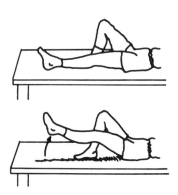

Knee Extension—Active

Stand with back against wall. Slide bottom down until knees are bent halfway.
Hold _____ counts.
Repeat _____ times.

Knee Extension—Quad Set

Lie on back, press _____ knee into mat, tightening muscle on front of thigh. Do not hold breath.
Hold _____ counts.
Repeat _____ times.

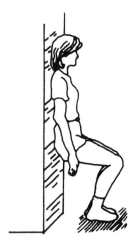

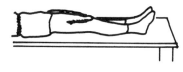

Knee Flexion—Stretching
Lie on back, towel roll under lower
back. Grasp right thigh with hands.
Try to straighten knee. Do not move
hip. Stretch is felt in back of thigh.
Hold _____ counts/minutes.
Repeat to left leg and hold.
Repeat _____ times.

Knee Flexion—Stretching
Lie on back, towel roll under lower
back. Place sheet around left foot.
Raise leg up with sheet. Keep knee
straight. Stretch is felt in back of thigh.
Hold _____ counts/minutes.
Repeat to right leg and hold.
Repeat _____ times.

Knee Flexion—Stretching   ✔
Sit with right leg off mat. Lean
forward, reaching for toes. Keep back
straight. Stretch is felt in back of thigh.
Hold _____ counts/minutes.
Repeat to opposite side and hold.
Repeat _____ times.

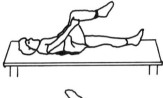
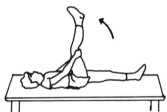
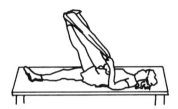
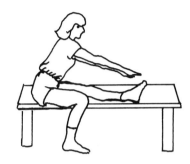

Knee Flexion—Stretching
Heel of right foot on step with toes up.
Lean forward, bending at hips. Keep
back straight. Stretch is felt in back of
thigh.
Hold _____ counts.
Repeat to left leg and hold.
Repeat _____ times.

Knee Extension—Stretching   ✔
Standing, hold onto table. Grasp
_____ ankle. Pull foot to bottom.
Stretch is felt in front of thigh.
Do not lean forward.
Hold _____ counts.
Repeat _____ times.
Progress to moving hip backward
with exercise.

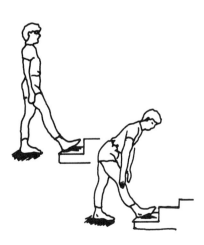
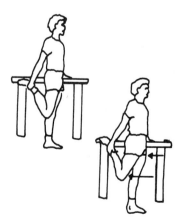

FCA Summary Letter

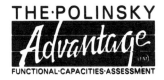

THE·POLINSKY
Advantage (TM)
FUNCTIONAL·CAPACITIES·ASSESSMENT

FCA SUMMARY LETTER

NAME: Doe, John
ADDRESS: 530 East 2nd Street
                Duluth, MN 55802
BIRTH DATE: 12/15/56
DIAGNOSIS: Lumbosacral strain
DATES OF FCA: 02/12/90, 02/13/90
PHYSICIAN: B. Stevens, M.D.

I.   John Doe has completed a standard Polinsky Functional
     Capacities Assessment and viewed an educational videotape on
     body mechanics.

II. Client worked to full capacity for all test items; therefore,
     the findings of this FCA are a valid picture of the client's
     maximum safe capabilities and limitations.

III. SIGNIFICANT FINDINGS FROM THE POLINSKY FCA PRELIMINARY
     ASSESSMENT

     A. Decreased trunk flexibility
     B. Rigid posture
     C. Increased thoracic and paraspinal muscle tightness

IV. THE FOLLOWING IS A SUMMARY OF THE OBJECTIVE FINDINGS AS
     PERFORMED BY THE CLIENT ON 02/12/90 AND 02/13/90.

     A. WEIGHT CAPACITIES:
        1. Level Lift   40 lbs.
        2. Weight Carry   40 lbs.
        3. Stand-up Lift   25 lbs.
        4. Overhead Lift   20 lbs.
        5. Unilateral Carry   25 lbs.   RIGHT
        6. Push   95 lbs.
        7. Pull   115 lbs.

     B. ACTIVITIES PERFORMED ADEQUATELY:
        1. Repeated Reciprocal Leg Motion
        2. Standing
        3. Walking
        4. Sitting
        5. Stairs
        6. Ladder
        7. Balance
        8. Left Hand Strength
        9. Right Hand Strength
        10. Left Upper Extremity Coordination
        11. Right Upper Extremity Coordination

#1102   Doe, John

C. MAJOR LIMITING FACTORS:

1. Decreased trunk strength and stability
2. Decreased lower extremity strength and endurance
3. Decreased upper extremity strength and endurance
4. Decreased trunk flexibility
5. Paraspinal muscle tightness
6. Complaints of discomfort in mid and low back

D. ACTIVITIES PERFORMED WITH FUNCTIONAL LIMITATIONS: (The numbers
correspond with the limiting factors listed above.)
1. Kneeling (1,5,6)
2. Unloaded Repeated Bending (4,5,6)
3. Overhead Reach Unweighted (1,3,6)
4. Overhead Reach Weighted (1,3,6)
5. Unloaded Rep. Squat (1,2,6)

E. ACTIVITIES UNABLE TO PERFORM: (The numbers
correspond with the limiting factors listed above.)
No activities.

F. ACTIVITIES SELF-LIMITED: (The numbers
correspond with the limiting factors listed above.)
No activities.

G. MAJOR STRENGTHS:

1. Good knowledge of body mechanics
2. Good upper extremity coordination
3. Good sitting and walking tolerance; adequate standing
   tolerance
4. Good use of relaxation techniques

V.   PHYSICAL AND OCCUPATIONAL THERAPY SUMMARY

The client understood that the purpose of the FCA was to find
the capabilities and limitations as they relate to work,
recreation, and activities of daily living.

A. COOPERATION

Client is a pleasant and cooperative individual. He reports
following a strengthening exercise program at home. He is
realistic as to what he can and cannot do, and although cautious
at the start of an activity, is willing to work to his maximum.
He has a positive outlook overall.

#1102   Doe, John

B. PAIN BEHAVIOR

   Client demonstrates minimal pain behaviors in the form of
   occasional facial grimaces and rubbing the low back. He
   complains of increased low back pain primarily when assuming
   forward or extended trunk positions and with increased weight
   loads on the lifts. He talked about pain only when specifically
   asked.

C. PACE, ENDURANCE, QUALITY OF MOTION

   Client works at an overall moderate pace. He uses smooth,
   efficient movements allowing an economy of motion, with the
   exception of forward bending and unloaded repeated squatting.
   He paces himself effectively during the FCA to allow maximum
   tolerance of each activity. Decreased upper extremity and
   lower extremity endurance was noted with overhead work and
   unloaded repeated squatting.

D. BODY MECHANICS; SAFETY AND WORK EFFICIENCY

   Client demonstrates he was able to perform activities with
   proper and safe body mechanics with minimal instruction. He
   required instructions to safely perform the push activity. He
   was instructed to ease into the push avoiding jerking motions,
   thus avoiding an increase in low back symptoms. Client was
   receptive to suggestions regarding exercise, body mechanics, and
   use of long-handled tools.

E. ABILITY TO COMPLETE TASKS

   Client adequately completed all activities of the Polinsky FCA,
   with the exception of kneeling, overhead work, unloaded
   repeated bending and unloaded repeated squatting due to the
   limiting factors as listed above.

F. CONSISTENCY

   Client was consistent Day 1 to Day 2 working to his maximum
   capacity. He complained of increased low and mid-back
   discomfort following Day 1 activities, but this did not affect
   his Day 2 performance. Client tolerated slightly increased
   weight loads, worked at a brisker pace, and was more at ease
   with assessment protocol on Day 2.

G. STATEMENT OF RELIABILITY BASED ON CLIENT'S PERFORMANCE

   There was good correlation between the preliminary assessment
   and all 20 activities of the Polinsky FCA, thus indicating a
   reliable result.

#1102   Doe, John

H. PRESENT ABILITIES COMPARED TO NORMING POPULATION

When comparing this client to normal, uninjured men his age who
have performed the FCA, he is an average performer for all
activities with the exception of the following: He is a less
than average performer for weight carry(time), weighted overhead
reach, balance C(errors), and balance C,D(time). He is a low
performer for the level lift, weight carry(lbs), stand-up lift,
kneeling, unloaded repeated bending and squatting, unweighted
overhead reach, and bilateral upper extremity coordination. It
is significant to note that the client is also functionally
limited in all of the less than average and low performance
activities. Performance on these activities also correlates
positively with the client's major limiting factors.

I. RECOMMENDED JOB CLASSIFICATION EXERTIONAL LEVEL

Client is capable of performing medium work. The regulations
define medium work as lifting/carrying no more than 50 pounds
at a time, with frequent lifting/carrying up to 25 pounds.
Being able to do frequent lifting/carrying up to 25 pounds is
often more critical than being able to lift up to 50 pounds at
a time. The considerable lifting required for the full range
of medium work usually requires frequent bending/stooping.

Standing/walking is generally required off and on for a total
of approximately 6 hours of an 8-hour workday. Sitting may
occur intermittently during the remaining 2 hours. In most
medium jobs, being on one's feet for most of the workday is
critical.

Medium work jobs require use of the arms and hands to grasp,
hold and turn objects but generally do not require the use of
fingers for fine activities to the extent required for
sedentary work.

To determine the physical exertion requirements of work in the
national economy, jobs are classified as "sedentary", "light",
"medium", "heavy", and "very heavy". These terms have the same
meaning as they have in the Dictionary of Occupational Titles,
published by the Department of Labor (Section 404.1567 and
416.967 of the Regulations).

VI. PHYSICAL AND OCCUPATIONAL THERAPY RECOMMENDATIONS

In reviewing the assessment, the need for the following general
recommendations is noted:

A. HOME PROGRAMS NEEDED

  1. Review stretching and strengthening exercises client is

- 4 -

#1102   Doe, John

presently doing at home. Assess the need for adding to or
modifying these exercises. Educate in additional activity
to increase trunk flexibility and decrease upper back
tightness.

2. Recommend instruction in abdominal, trunk and leg
strengthening exercises.

3. Encourage activities such as walking, riding a stationary
bike or swimming for overall strengthening and conditioning.

B. RETURN TO WORK

A job description was not provided. Client is a diesel mechanic
which, he reports, involves heavy lifting and not much bending,
twisting, climbing, working from a ladder, pushing or overhead
work. He is able to lift and carry 25 lbs. frequently, and push
and pull occasionally. He is limited in overhead reach work to
an occasional basis when weight is involved. Client stated he
could work on smaller engines as the average lifting required
is approximately 25-35 lbs. He reported he would have minimal
difficulty returning to work on this basis. This therapist
would be willing to assist if asked for input regarding
specific job activities.

C. APPROPRIATE REFERRALS

A work hardening program is recommended if client is unable to
return to work per FCA guidelines. Specific goals for work
hardening would be to increase weight capacities to the level
needed to return to work, increase ability to tolerate static
weight-bearing activities (specifically kneeling and standing),
increase trunk flexibility, and increase tolerance of overhead
work positions. Retest weighted activities and functionally
limited areas following work hardening to assess gains.

_____

Mary Johnson, PT
Physical Therapist

_____

Alice Meyer, OTR
Occupational Therapist

cc: B. Stevens, M.D.
     Daniel John, QRC

Client Name: Doe, John   Client #:   1102
Age: 33   Male

FCA Items	FCA Test Results	FCA Normal Data Comparison*	N	OC	FREQ	CONT	Exertion Level
1. Level Lift	40	LOW	>41	27 - 40	11 - 26	1 - 10	M
2. Weight Carry	40	LOW	>41	27 - 40	11 - 26	1 - 10	M
Time	00:35	LAP					
3. Stand-Up Lift	25	LOW	>26	17 - 25	7 - 16	1 - 6	M
4. Kneeling	06:00	LOW					
5. Unload. Rep. Bend	12/min	LOW					
Time	02:48	LOW					
6. Overhead Lift	20		>21	14 - 20	6 - 13	1 - 5	M
7. Unilat. Carry	25		>26	17 - 25	7 - 16	1 - 6	M
Time	00:38						
8. Push	95	AP			X		
9. Pull	115	AP			X		
10. Rep. Recip. Leg	10:00	AP				X	
11. OH Reach Wghtd	02:10	LAP		X			
OH Reach Unwghtd	05:05	LOW		X			
12. Standing	35:00	AP			X		M
13. Walking	50/100	AP			X		M
Time	09:30	AP					
14. Sitting	30:00	AP				X	M
15. Stairs	75/min	AP			X		
Time	04:00	AP					
16. Ladder	ABLE	AP			X		
17. Balance							
(a) time	00:28	AP					
errors	0	AP				X	
(b) time	00:50	AP					
errors	0	AP					
(c) time	01:28	LAP					
errors	2	LAP					
(d) time	00:38	LAP					
errors	0	AP					
18. Unload. Rep Squat	10/min	LOW		X			
time	01:58	LOW					
19. Hand Strength							
right	92	AP			X		
left	85	AP			X		
20. U/E Coordination							
right	93	LOW				X	
left	94	LOW				X	

* AA = above average performance   (+1 SD above mean)
   AP = average performance   (-1 SD below mean)
   LAP = less than average   (-1 to -2 below mean)
   LOW = low performance   (more than -2 SD below mean)

** OC   = occasionally   65-100% of maximum   (1-33% of day)
   FREQ = frequently   25-64% of maximum   (34-66% of day)
   CONT = continuously   1-25% of maximum   (67-100% of day)
   N   = never
   Percentages are suggested guidelines used to compute 1, 2, 3, 6, and 7

Workers' Compensation Administration Directory

The Workers' Compensation Directory is provided as a convenience to readers who wish to obtain copies of relevant state regulations.

WORKER'S COMPENSATION ADMINISTRATION DIRECTORY

ALABAMA

Workmen's Compensation
ATTN: Harold Walker
P.O. Box 12046
Birmingham, AL 35202-2046

ALASKA

Workmen's Compensation Division
Department of Labor
P.O. Box 25512
Juneau, AK 99802
(907) 465-2790

ARIZONA

Industrial Commission
800 West Washington
P.O. Box 19070
Phoenix, AZ 85005-9070
(602) 542-4661

ARKANSAS

**Worker's Compensation
Commission**
625 Marshall Street
Justice Building
Little Rock, AR 72201
(501) 682-3930

CALIFORNIA

Workers' Compensation
Division of Industrial Accidents
395 Oyster Point Boulevard
South San Francisco, CA 94080
(415) 737-2610

COLORADO

Workers' Compensation Board
1120 Lincoln
Denver, CO 80203
(303) 764-2929
(303) 866-2782

CONNECTICUT

Workers' Compensation Commission
1890 Dixwell Avenue
Hamden, CT 06514
(203) 789-7783

DELAWARE

Industrial Accident Board
State Office Building
Sixth Floor
820 North French Street
Wilmington, DE 19801
(302) 577-2885

DISTRICT OF COLUMBIA

Department of Employment Services
Office of Workers' Compensation
P.O. Box 56098
Washington, DC 20011
(202) 576-6265

FLORIDA

Division of Workers' Compensation
301 Forest Building
2728 Centerview Drive
Tallahassee, FL 32399-0680
(904) 488-2548

GEORGIA

Board of Workers' Compensation
Suite 1000, South Tower
One CNN Center
Atlanta, GA 30303-2788
(404) 656-3875

HAWAII

Disability Compensation Division
Department of Labor and Industrial Relations
830 Punchbowl Street, Room 209
Honolulu, HI 96813
(808) 548-4131

IDAHO

Workers' Compensation
1215 W. State Street
Boise, ID 83720
(208) 334-2470

ILLINOIS

Workers' Compensation Industrial Commission
100 W. Randolf
Chicago, IL 60601
(312) 814-6500

INDIANA

Workers' Compensation
402 W. Washington Street
Room W196
Indiana Government Center South
Indianapolis, IN 46204
(317) 232-3808

IOWA

Industrial Commissioner's Office
1000 E. Grand Avenue
Des Moines, IA 50319
(515) 281-5935

KANSAS

Division of Workers' Compensation: Rehab Division
800 South West Jackson
600 Merchants Bank Tower
Topeka, KS 66612-1276
(913) 296-2050

KENTUCKY

Workers' Compensation Board
Perimeter Park West
Building C
1270 Louisville Road
Frankfort, KY 40601
(502) 564-5550

LOUISIANA

Department of Labor
Office of Workers' Compensation
P.O. Box 94040
Baton Rouge, LA 70804-9040
(504) 342-7555

MAINE

**Workers' Compensation
Commission**
State House Station 27
State Office Building
Augusta, ME 04333
(207) 289-3751

MARYLAND

**Workmen's Compensation
Commission**
6 North Liberty Street
Baltimore, MD 21201
(301) 333-4700

NEW HAMPSHIRE

Department of Labor
State Office Park South
95 Pleasant Street
Concord, NH 03301
(603) 271-3171

NEW JERSEY

**Division of Workers'
Compensation**
John Fitch Plaza
Call Number 381
Trenton, NJ 08625
(609) 292-2414

NEW MEXICO

**Workers' Compensation
Administration**
P.O. Box 27198
Albuquerque, NM 87125-7198
(505) 841-6000

NEW YORK

Workers' Compensation Board
180 Livingston Street
Brooklyn, NY 11248
(718) 802-6600

NORTH CAROLINA

Industrial Commission
Dobbs Building
430 North Salisbury Street
Raleigh, NC 27611
(919) 733-4820

NORTH DAKOTA

Workmens' Compensation Bureau
Russell Building - Hwy 83 North
4007 N. State Street
Bismarck, ND 58501
(701) 224-3800

OHIO

**Bureau of Workers'
Compensation**
246 North High Street
Columbus, OH 43266-0581
(614) 466-2950

OKLAHOMA

Workers' Compensation Court
1915 N. Stiles
Oklahoma City, OK 73105
(405) 557-7600

OREGON

Workers' Compensation Board
480 Church Street Northeast
Salem, OR 97310
(503) 378-3308

MASSACHUSETTS

Industrial Accident Board
600 Washington Street
Boston, MA 02111
(617) 727-4900

MICHIGAN

**Bureau of Workers' Disability
Compensation**
Department of Labor
P.O. Box 30016
Victor Building, 2nd Floor
201 North Washington Square
Lansing, MI 48909
(517) 373-3480

MINNESOTA

Workers' Compensation Division
Department of Labor & Industry
444 Lafayette Road
St. Paul, MN 55101
(612) 296-2432

MISSISSIPPI

**Workmen's Compensation
Commission**
1428 Lakeland Drive
P.O. Box 5300
Jackson, MS 39296-5300
(601) 987-4200

MISSOURI

**Division of Workers'
Compensation**
*Department of Labor
and Industrial Relations*
P.O. Box 58
Jefferson City, MO 65102
(314) 751-4231

MONTANA

**State Compensation
Mutual Insurance Fund**
Division of Workers' Compensation
5 South Last Chance Gulch
P.O. Box 4759
Helena, MT 59604
(406) 444-6518

NEBRASKA

Workmen's Compensation Court
Lincoln, NE 68509-8908
(402) 471-2568

NEVADA

State Industrial Insurance System
515 East Musser Street
Carson City, NV 89714
(702) 687-5220

PENNSYLVANIA

Bureau of Workers' Compensation
1171 South Cameron Street, Rm 103
Harrisburg, PA 17104-2501
(717) 783-5421

RHODE ISLAND

Department of Workers' Compensation
610 Manton Avenue
Providence, RI 02909
(401) 272-0700

SOUTH CAROLINA

Workers' Compensation Commission
P.O. Box 1715
Columbia, SC 29202-1715
(803) 737-5700

SOUTH DAKOTA

Division of Labor and Management
Kneip Building
700 Governors Drive
Pierre, SD 57501-2291
(605) 773-3681

TENNESSEE

Department of Labor Tennessee W/C Division
501 Union Building, 2nd Floor
Nashville, TN 37243-0661
(615) 741-2395

TEXAS

Texas W/C Commission
4000 South IH35
Austin, TX 78704
(512) 448-7900

UTAH

W/C Fund of Utah
P.O. Box 45420
Salt Lake City, UT 84145-0420
(801) 538-8000

VERMONT

Department of Labor & Industry
Workers' Compensation Division
120 State Street
Montpelier, VT 05620
(802) 828-2286

VIRGINIA

Industrial Commission of Virginia
P.O. Box 1794
Richmond, VA 23214
(804) 367-8600

WASHINGTON

Department of Labor & Industries
Claims Division HC-242
Olympia, WA 98504
(206) 753-6341

WEST VIRGINIA

West Virginia Workers' Compensation
P.O. Box 3151
Charleston, WV 25332
(304) 348-3423

WISCONSIN

Department of Industry, Labor & Human Relations
Workers' Compensation Division
P.O. Box 7901
Madison, WI 53707
(608) 266-1340

WYOMING

Workers' Compensation Division
122 West 25th Street, 2nd Floor
East Wing, Herschler Building
Cheyenne, WY 82002
(800) 228-6194

Product Vendors

Antivibration Gloves
   Malcolm G. Stevens, Inc.
   P.O. Box 145
   Arlington, MA 02174
   (Steel Grip, Inc.)
   (617) 648-4112

CARF Guidelines
   CARF
   101 North Wilmot Road
   Suite 500
   Tucson, AZ 85711

Cervical Pillows Physiotechnology, Inc.
   1925 West 6th Street
   Topeka, KS 66606
   (800) 255-3554

Chatillon Dynamometer
   State Scales Company, Inc.
   155 Bemis Road, RFD 12
   Manchester, NH 03102
   (603) 625-8274

Ergonomic Supplies
   North Coast Medical, Inc.
   187 Stauffer Boulevard
   San Jose, CA 95125-1042
   (800) 821-9319

Figure 8 Posture Braces
Tennis Elbow Splints
   Freeman Manufacturing Company
   900 West Chicago Road
   Drawer J
   Sturgis, MI 49091
   (800) 253-2091

Hand Grippers
   Tafco Manufacturing Company
   15220 SE Meadowlark Lane
   Portland, OR 97222
   (503) 654-3549

LMB Splint
   LMB Hand Rehab Products, Inc.
   P.O. Box 1181
   San Luis Obispo, CA 93406-1181

Lumbar Rolls and Pillows
   Bird and Cronin
   2601 East 80th Street
   Minneapolis, MN 55420
   (800) 328-1095

   Medic-Air Corp of America
   16 North Chatsworth Avenue
   Larchmont, NY 10538

Myoflex Analgesic Creme
   Rorer Consumer Pharmaceuticals
   500 Virginia Drive
   Fort Washington, PA 19034
   (800) 221-1066

Progressive Individualized Exercises
   Joelle Schneider, Joan Carol Cecil
   Therapy Skill Builders
   3830 East Bellevue
   P.O. Box 42050
   Tucson, AZ 85733
   (602) 323-7500

Viscolas Shoe Inserts Back Books
Sex and Back Pain Books
   IMPACC
   89 Hillside Avenue
   Bangor, ME 04401
   (207) 941-0290

Volumeter
   Volumeters Unlimited
   52421 Double View Drive
   P.O. Box 146
   Idyllwild, CA 92349
   (714) 659-2619

"Your Healthy Upper Body School" Blueprints:
   Ergocrate, Ergosled, and Ergostation
Slide Marketing Package Work Hardening Orientation
   Booklets
   Ergonomics Plus—
   A Division of MPTC
   P.O. Box 1450
   Scarborough, ME 04070-1450
   (207) 883-3406
   (207) 883-3454 FAX

INDEX